THE WOMAN'S DAY
WEIGHT-LOSS PLAN

THE WOMAN'S DAY WEIGHT-LOSS PLAN

LOSE WEIGHT
EAT RIGHT
BE FIT *and*
FEEL GREAT *at*
EVERY STAGE *of* LIFE!

KATHY KEENAN ISOLDI, M.S., R.D., C.D.E.

filipacchi publishing

Woman's Day

CREDITS

Breakfast Smoothie: Crate & Barrel "Simon" glass mug and "Clio" footed glass.

Herb and Avocado Canapés: Villeroy & Boch "New Wave" square white bowl.

Pan-Fried Pork Chops: Crate & Barrel "Ovation" flatware.

Broiled Salmon: Crate & Barrel "Vario" plate and Matchstick Brown mat.

Apricot-Lemon Glazed Fish Fillets: Villeroy & Boch "City Life" plate.

Chicken Vegetable Stir-Fry: Mariposa "Spiaggia" plate and bowl and Crate & Barrel Matchstick Natural mat.

Bow-Tie Pasta: Crate & Barrel "Elements" bowl.

Tangy Tuna Salad: Crate & Barrel "Luna" green bowl, board and white bowl, "Pleats" flatware.

Lentils with a Twist: Crate & Barrel "Serena" bowl.

Green Beans with Chive Cream Sauce: Villeroy & Boch "Palm" bowls and Crate & Barrel Circle Orange mat.

Tangy Vinaigrette Dressing: Crate & Barrel "Conical Individual" glass bowl.

Apple and Pear Parfait: Crate & Barrel "Strap Green" mat.

Crate & Barrel: *www.crateandbarrel.com.* For a store near you, call 800-996-9960.

Mariposa: *www.mariposa.com.* For a store near you, call 800-996-9960.

Villeroy & Boch: *www.villeroy-boch.com.* For a store near you, call 800-VILLEROY.

To my husband Fred, whose love and encouragement knows no end, and who inspires me every day; and to my children, Michelle, Brian and Gregory, who fill my life with immense happiness, and selflessly offer their love and support while I write.

Filipacchi Publishing
1633 Broadway
New York, NY 10019

© 2003 Filipacchi Publishing
Interior photographs © 2003 Jacqueline Hopkins
Jacket photographs: Jacqueline Hopkins (food);
    Jenny Acheson

Designed by Patricia Fabricant
Edited by Madonna Behen

ISBN 2-85018-645-7

Manufactured in the United States of America

CONTENTS

Foreword

BY LOUIS J. ARONNE, M.D.

A S I'M SURE YOU'RE WELL AWARE, the incidence of overweight and obesity in this country is rising at an alarming rate. This rise greatly concerns those of us in the health care community, because so many serious illnesses are triggered or exacerbated by carrying around excess pounds. Of particular concern is the link between being overweight and the increased risk of developing three diseases that take the lives of many women each year: heart disease, diabetes and certain forms of cancer. Fortunately, overweight women can reduce their risk of developing these chronic, life-threatening health problems by losing just 5 to 10 percent of their body weight.

While both men and women suffer from the ill effects of being overweight, women carry the unique burden of trying to maintain a healthy weight while managing a lifetime of physical changes. Hormonal shifts can increase appetite, and pregnancy may cause women to deposit fat with greater ease. Menopause is also a particularly difficult time to try to lose weight. In addition, I find that the women I see in my office juggle many responsibilities, including parenting, homemaking and career. All these tasks can keep them from eating right and exercising as much as they know they should.

Maintaining a healthy weight can be a challenge for many women, but the health benefits of winning the war on weight are well worth the fight. To win, you don't have to lose enough weight to fit back into your prom dress or achieve a weight lower than you've ever been as an adult. Success is attained by setting your sights on a healthy weight—one that you can achieve and maintain. By the same token, successfully incorporating more physical activity into your life doesn't mean you have to join a gym and pump iron seven days a week. Being more physically active now, a year from now and five years from now because you planned a realistic exercise regimen is the real measure of success.

Following a diet you can continue long-term is another key to weight-loss success. Diets that promise you'll be a new person in two quick weeks just won't work. And investing your time, energy and hopes into diet plans that can't work creates a vicious cycle of failure that will leave you feeling defeated and that will set you up for gaining more weight than you've lost.

What you need to succeed is a realistic plan that meets your nutritional needs and is based on the latest scientific research—just like the plan outlined in this book, designed by Kathy Keenan Isoldi, M.S., R.D., C.D.E., my colleague at the Comprehensive Weight Control Program in New York City.

Kathy and I have worked together for fifteen years, helping thousands of patients fight the good fight in the war on weight. When Kathy came to work with me, she already had seven years of patient care and experience under her belt. Her years of experience are matched by her caring nature and deep level of understanding of the plight of her patients. This level of caring, along with a passion for improving the health of her patients, is what drives her to find solutions to the many obstacles our patients face. And that's why so many patients put their trust in her and why they find success and contentment in the plan she designs.

I can see Kathy's unique architectural blueprints on every page of this book. Her kind and caring voice bounces right off the pages to guide you though the program, to help you along with suggestions to overcome challenges and to encourage you to persevere. I wish you well in your quest to lose weight, increase your physical activity and improve your health. You have so much to gain by losing weight!

DR. LOUIS ARONNE, a nationally-known obesity expert, is a clinical associate professor of medicine at Weill Medical College of Cornell University in New York City. He is also the founder and director of the Comprehensive Weight Control Program, a multidisciplinary obesity research and treatment center.

Introduction

WHY IS IT SO HARD FOR WOMEN to maintain a healthy weight? Let me count the ways: stress, lack of time, childbirth and lactation, caring for children, job-related responsibilities, stress, maintaining a romantic relationship, lack of time, caring for aging parents, stress, menopause, lack of time and stress. You get the picture: stress and lack of time are constant obstacles to caring for yourself. Juggling all those balls at once takes its toll, and the end product is often weight gain.

Close to 50 percent of American women are overweight or obese. Unhealthy weight gain is also associated with an increased risk of developing eight life-threatening illnesses. It's a sad but true fact that 300,000 Americans die each year because of obesity-related complications. Overweight and obesity are increasing at an alarming annual rate, and experts predict that obesity will soon surpass cigarette smoking as the number-one preventable cause of death in the United States.

Making the decision to get in shape is empowering and lifesaving, and it's the first step in taking proper care of yourself. Women have traditionally been socialized to care for others and, in the process, many lose sight of the need to care for themselves. Unfortunately, at a time when many women are looking to improve their health by losing weight, they are bombarded with countless options and opinions on weight loss. The problem is that all the weight-loss information out there is not necessarily valid, useful or true. You know the saying, "If it sounds too good to be true, it probably is." This warning rings especially true when it comes to evaluating weight-loss promises.

I understand that if you hear the claim "lose 30 pounds in 30 days," your ears will perk up. However, examine the promise carefully. Is there scientific research behind it or just reports of success from individuals? What is the quality of the research? If it is a truly groundbreaking, scientifically proven obesity treatment, the news will be plastered across newspaper front pages and reported on the major television networks. Also, consider whether the diet plan will promote health as well as weight loss. Some plans that exclude entire food groups deprive your body of essential nutrients, ones that have been found to decrease the risk of major illnesses. Ask yourself, "Can I follow this plan for life?" Many of my patients report having some success with fad diets, but then tell me they couldn't follow the rigid guidelines for extended periods of time.

The *Woman's Day* weight-loss plan outlined in this book was created using the most up-to-date scientific research data available on weight loss and disease prevention. So when you hop aboard this program, what you'll get is a plan for eating and exercising that's realistic and healthy, that will allow you to lose weight without feeling hungry and that you can follow forever!

We've also made this diet and exercise plan extremely woman-friendly by including sections that address your age-specific needs. Women encounter unique challenges at each stage of life. This book takes you through these stages with solutions that you can use right away. Instead of hitting roadblocks that interfere with your plan to eat right and exercise, you will face each day with practical solutions to overcome these obstacles.

The book begins with a review of the health risks of obesity and how you can improve your health with weight loss. This is followed by the "nuts and bolts" of the diet plan, which is outlined in a clear and easy-to-understand manner. We've provided exercise guidance, lots of healthy recipes and thirty days of menus to help you get started right away. Worksheets offer additional guidance in planning and maintaining your new way of life.

The main section of the book addresses the various stages of a woman's life, beginning with the early days of college and dating, through marriage and motherhood and ending with menopause and beyond. Regardless of the stage of life you're at when you begin this plan, you will find success. You may also want to share this book with the women in your life who are also struggling with weight problems.

Now, let's begin taking care of the woman who takes care of everyone else and start you on a plan for health, empowerment and weight loss.

PART ONE

Knowledge Is Power

1. Weighty Issues for Women

LIVING A LONGER, HEALTHIER LIFE

IN THE EARLY 1900S, women had an average lifespan of 48 years. With improvements in health care and quality of life, we've been able to add about three decades to that number. While complications of childbirth, tuberculosis and infection were the demons plaguing women of yesteryear, the risks facing women in the twenty-first century are much different. Ask women what their health concerns are, and you'll hear that cancer, especially breast cancer, is a major worry. Many also see their moms suffering with the disabilities brought on by osteoarthritis and wonder if this disease is in their own future. While heart disease, diabetes and high blood pressure are serious illnesses, women often don't worry about them as much as they should.

It's estimated that more than 300,000 Americans die each year due to complications from obesity-related illnesses. The good news is that losing even a small amount of weight can dramatically improve your health and reduce your risk of developing these illnesses. Even if you already suffer from a weight-related illness, weight loss will undoubtedly improve your health. Many diabetics and those suffering from high blood pressure are able to reduce, or sometimes even eliminate, medication when they lose weight. This process requires your doctor's guidance and a lot of monitoring, but wouldn't it be wonderful if you were able to reduce your need for medication while losing weight? You can achieve all of this—live longer, be healthier, reduce your risk of developing illness and reduce the severity of any of your existing weight-related diseases—with healthy changes in your diet and lifestyle.

The risk of cardiovascular disease (including heart disease, stroke and high blood pressure), diabetes, cancer, osteoarthritis, respiratory illnesses and gallbladder disease all increase in women as weight rises. Two other conditions—metabolic syndrome (also known as syndrome X) and polycystic ovary syndrome (PCOS)—warrant discussion, as well, since more women are diagnosed with these puzzling weight-related syndromes every day.

CARDIOVASCULAR DISEASE

MORE WOMEN DIE FROM CARDIOVASCULAR DISEASE than from all forms of cancer combined. It accounts for about half of all female deaths, taking the lives of almost 500,000 women each year. About half of that total, or 250,000 women, die every year due to heart disease alone. Women are hit hardest with cardiovascular disease after the age of 65 (about a decade later than men). However, more than 20,000 women under the age of 65 die of heart attacks each year.

Polls report that most women are unaware of how life-threatening heart disease can be. A 2002 report found that only about 20 percent of women interviewed were aware that cardiovascular disease is the major cause of death in women. This lack of awareness may prevent women from taking corrective, aggressive action to reduce the risk of this mighty killer. It's always sad to hear a woman say, "If I had only known, I would have paid more attention to my diet and exercise in the past." Now you are a woman in the know. Cardiovascular disease is a woman's disease, it's a deadly disease and you can intercept its progress by making changes in your diet and lifestyle.

Risk Factors for Heart Disease

Coronary artery disease is often caused by the accumulation of plaque in the vessels leading to the heart. Plaque buildup, also known as atherosclerosis, narrows the vessels and impedes blood flow. If plaque obstructs the blood flow completely, a heart attack occurs. While there are certain risks to developing heart disease that you don't have control over—such as your family history, age and genetics—there are plenty of risk factors that you can modify, such as weight gain and eating a high-fat diet.

Heart Disease and Women	
RISK FACTOR	ACTIONS THAT LOWER RISK
Smoking	• Don't start smoking. • Stop smoking if you do smoke.
Diabetes	• Monitor and work on lowering blood sugar readings. • Exercise, which has been shown to lower blood glucose readings. • Lose weight if you are overweight or obese.
Hypertension	• Take any prescribed medication. • Monitor blood pressure readings. • Engage in moderate exercise, which helps to lower blood pressure. • Limit sodium and include foods rich in magnesium, calcium and potassium.*
Obesity	• Achieve and maintain a healthy weight through reduced calorie intake and increased exercise.
High blood lipid levels**	• Decrease intake of saturated fat, trans-fatty acids and cholesterol. • Eat more fiber-rich and whole-grain foods. • Eat more food high in omega-3 fatty acids.[†] • Exercise.

*   Dairy products, fruits, vegetables and beans.
** High lipid levels refer to all different types of fat in your blood. Cholesterol is one fat in your bloodstream that increases your risk of cardiovascular disease, but there are other lipids (or fats) in your bloodstream that contribute to plaque formation. (See page 16 for more information).
[†]   Omega-3 fatty acids are found in salmon, tuna and canola oil.

HYPERTENSION

Many people carrying around extra weight stress their system, and it shows up in increased blood pressure readings. Those who are overweight or obese are two to three times more likely to develop high blood pressure than people who maintain a healthy weight. While elevated blood pressure is not always caused by weight gain, it's thought to be a contributing factor in about half of Caucasians and a quarter of African Americans.

Normal blood pressure readings measure 120/80 or lower. Any reading of 130 to 139/85 to 89 is considered borderline hypertension, and 140/90 or higher is classified as high blood pressure. If you have an above-average blood pressure reading, it is essential that you monitor your blood pressure and discuss all treatment options with your doctor. Untreated blood pressure can lead to heart disease, kidney disease or stroke.

DIABETES MELLITUS, TYPE 2

Type 2 diabetes is on the rise in epidemic proportions. About 6.5 million women in the U.S. have Type 2 diabetes, and half of them don't know it. There is a definite link between weight gain and the development of this disease. Results from the ongoing Nurses' Health Study show that women with a body mass index over 35 have a 60 times greater risk of developing diabetes than women in the lowest weight group.

There is definitely a genetic component to developing Type 2 diabetes, and having had gestational diabetes places you at increased risk, too. If diabetes runs in your family and/or you have a history of gestational diabetes and you're overweight, losing weight and changing your diet to a low glycemic plan (see Chapter 2), will help prevent this illness.

Unlike people with Type 1 diabetes, those with Type 2 do produce insulin, the hormone that transports glucose (sugar) from the bloodstream across cell membranes to be used for energy. The problem is that, in Type 2 diabetes, the cells will not accept the insulin that's available. In the face of this insulin resistance, the pancreas pumps out more and more insulin in an attempt to lower elevated blood glucose levels. Eventually, the cells accept the insulin (sometimes all at once), causing blood sugar levels to plummet. Even if you don't have diabetes, insulin resistance followed by excessive release of more insulin causes peaks and valleys in sugar levels, and the valleys cause low blood sugar reactions including increased hunger, headache, fatigue and heightened food cravings. This, of course, sets you up for overeating and weight gain, which increases your risk of developing Type 2 diabetes.

Experts believe that insulin resistance is a precursor to the diagnosis of Type 2 diabetes by anywhere from five to ten years. Over time, the overworked pancreas secretes less insulin, or secretes insulin too late, and diabetes develops. Weight loss and eating a healthy diet (rich in fiber and whole grains, with limits on white-flour carbohydrates) is your best shot at protection against this deadly illness. If you already have Type 2 diabetes,

Blood Lipid Levels: What Does It All Mean?

FAT (LIPID)	DEFINITION	FOUND IN THE FOLLOWING FOODS	NORMAL BLOOD RANGES*
Cholesterol	A fat-like substance produced by animals (in the liver), necessary in small amounts. However, excess levels increase risk of heart disease.	Since cholesterol is only made by animals, it's only found in animal products such as meat, cheese and butter.	<200 milligrams
Triglyceride	A fat found in food and in your body. It's a combination of fat and glucose. Therefore, sugar-rich foods as well as fats can boost this fat in your blood to an unhealthy level.	High-fat foods, such as butter and cream cheese, and high-sugar foods, such as desserts and juices, will boost triglyceride levels. Alcohol will raise triglyceride levels, too.	<150 milligrams
High-density lipoprotein cholesterol (HDL)	A protein carrier for cholesterol. It transports cholesterol to the liver for excretion, therefore aiding in the removal of cholesterol from the body.	Monounsaturated fats in olive oil and almonds and walnuts have been found to help raise HDL levels. Exercise will help raise HDL levels.	>40 milligrams
Low-density lipoprotein cholesterol (LDL)	A protein carrier for cholesterol, it transports fat throughout the body. High LDL levels increase your risk of heart disease.	Saturated fats, such as full-fat dairy foods, baked goods with hydrogenated oils, and meat.	<100 milligrams

* These levels are ranges for adults.

weight loss will improve your health. In some cases, diabetes may actually go into remission. Chapter 2 provides guidelines for diabetics who want to follow the diet plan outlined in this book.

METABOLIC SYNDROME

An estimated 47 million Americans have the metabolic syndrome—a dangerous cluster of symptoms that can dramatically increase the risk of diabetes, high blood pressure, stroke and heart disease. As with Type 2 diabetes, the fuel driving this syndrome is insulin resistance. People who are hyperinsulinemic (meaning they have too much insulin circulating in their bloodstream) will often exhibit many abnormalities in their system (see box, *above*). But you need not exhibit every clinical sign to have the syndrome. Unfortunately, many doctors still miss diagnosing this syndrome, and some individuals may be misled into eating a very lowfat, high-carbohydrate diet in an attempt to lose weight and improve cholesterol levels. This kind of diet will only worsen insulin resistance by stimulating the pancreas to secrete more insulin.

While experts say a genetic predisposition is likely, it's weight gain and inactivity that bring this syndrome to life. So diet and exercise are the gold standard of care for this syndrome. A low glycemic diet like the one in this book will help to keep insulin levels down, although some patients also require medication to lower insulin levels. If you suspect you have metabolic syndrome, you should see an endocrinologist who has experience in treating patients with this illness.

> **THE SIGNS OF METABOLIC SYNDROME**
>
> - Elevated blood pressure readings
> - Obesity, especially around the abdomen
> - Elevated glucose readings
> - Low HDL (good) cholesterol levels
> - High triglyceride levels

POLYCYSTIC OVARY SYNDROME

Polycystic ovary syndrome (PCOS) was first identified in 1935, but many women today have never heard about it. PCOS is the most common endocrine disorder in women, affecting 5 to 10 percent of all women in their reproductive years. It's a leading cause of infertility, and it increases a woman's risk of developing diabetes, cardiovascular disease and endometrial cancer. Again, the underlying cause of the syndrome is a high insulin level. Most experts believe that there is a genetic component to this syndrome, since PCOS tends to run in families.

In PCOS, chronically elevated levels of luteinizing hormone (LH) and insulin work together to wreak havoc on the entire body, causing increased testosterone production and ovarian cyst formation. However, losing just

5 to 7 percent of body weight has been shown to reduce insulin and testosterone levels and improve HDL cholesterol and triglyceride readings. Here, again, reducing total calories, limiting carbohydrates and exercising have been shown to improve the health of women with PCOS. If you suspect you have this condition, you should seek help from an endocrinologist who has experience with PCOS, since medication or other treatments may be necessary.

CERTAIN CANCERS

There is a documented increased risk of cancer of the breast, endometrium, ovaries, colon and gallbladder with increased body weight. Again, too much insulin is believed to play a role in increasing the risk of these hormone-dependent cancers, mainly because insulin increases the levels of certain hormones that may stimulate tumor growth. In addition, being overweight or obese adversely affects breast and endometrial cancer risk in postmenopausal women by exposing tissues to higher estrogen levels. For these reasons, following a diet that reduces blood insulin levels and helps maintain a healthy body weight appears to be prudent.

OSTEOARTHRITIS

One in three women will suffer from osteoarthritis. While there are many risk factors for developing this disease, including increasing age, carrying around excessive weight is a strong risk factor that you can control. Every additional 10 pounds of body weight you carry adds 30 pounds of pressure on your joints when you walk. Some research suggests that vitamin C, beta-carotene and vitamin E may help reduce the pain of osteoarthritis.

GALLBLADDER DISEASE

Gallstones are more prevalent in women with body mass indexes (BMIs) over 30. A woman with a BMI over 35 increases fourfold her risk of developing painful gallstones than a woman with a BMI of 24. While losing weight will help you lower the risk of developing gallstones, if you already have them, you need to be careful not to lose weight too quickly. Rapid weight loss can actually precipitate a gallbladder attack, as the stones may increase in size. If you have been diagnosed with gallstones, be sure to discuss this risk with your doctor before starting a weight-loss plan.

SLEEP APNEA

Sleep apnea is a condition that causes people to momentarily stop breathing in their sleep repeatedly during the night. While the problem affects more men than women, it's commonly underdiagnosed in overweight and obese women. Left untreated, sleep apnea causes daytime exhaustion that can lead to overeating, drowsiness and an increase in accidents. Untreated sleep apnea is also believed to increase the risk of heart attack and stroke. Experts say even a 10-pound weight loss is often enough for people to see an improvement in their symptoms.

Sleep apnea occurs when an excess amount of tissue in the airway causes it to narrow, which prevents air from easily flowing into or out of the nose or mouth. This results in heavy snoring, periods of no breathing, and frequent arousals (causing abrupt changes from deep sleep to light sleep). It's often the significant other who is aware of the symptoms of sleep apnea. Drinking alcohol intensifies the frequency and duration of breathing pauses. If you suspect you have sleep apnea, you should speak with your doctor about being evaluated in a sleep study clinic for diagnosis and treatment.

2. Get Started Eating Right...Today

DIET PLANS THAT PROMISE QUICK FIXES for a problem as complex as obesity can mislead you into believing that losing weight is a "piece of cake." But to lose all the weight you need to, and to keep that weight off for good, takes a bit more effort. While you don't need to get an advanced degree in nutrition to succeed in losing weight, you do need to gain some practical knowledge about food and calories. This knowledge will provide you with the tools necessary to tackle all your food challenges, every day of the year.

HOW MANY CALORIES DO YOU NEED?

I HAVE MANY PATIENTS who know the calorie count of every food in their refrigerator, and yet have no idea how many calories they need to meet their daily needs, let alone how many they should eat to lose weight. In my mind, not knowing how many calories you need to consume to lose weight is comparable to signing a mortgage contract without knowing your yearly earnings. Your estimated calorie need is information you must have, and I'm going to show you how to do the math to get your vital statistics.

But first, it's helpful to know what, exactly, calories are. A calorie is a unit of energy. It provides your body with the fuel it needs to perform many different functions. Energy is extracted from the food you eat and is transferred, via enzymes, into the energy that is needed to pump your heart, work your lungs and to power your brain so you can read this chapter.

Scientists measure the calorie content of a food by placing it in an insulated chamber surrounded by water. The food source is then burned, and the surrounding water temperature is measured. It takes one calorie to raise one gram of water one degree centigrade. So, if the water temperature in the bomb calorimeter is raised 10 degrees centigrade when the food item is burned, it contains 10 calories.

Back in the early 1900s, J. Arthur Harris and Francis G. Benedict, two scientists at the Carnegie Institute of Washington in Boston, conducted research that laid the foundation for establishing calorie needs in humans, taking into account variables such as age, gender, height, weight and physical activity. Nearly a century later, the Harris-Benedict Formula continues to be used as an accurate yardstick for determining your body's basal metabolic rate (BMR)—the calorie level required to perform basic bodily functions.

THE BMR FORMULA FOR WOMEN

$$BMR = 655 + (4.3 \times weight) + (4.7 \times height) - (4.7 \times age)$$
IN POUNDS   IN INCHES   IN YEARS

Let's plug in the data for a woman we'll call Nancy. Nancy is 39 years old, 5'6" tall and weighs 190 pounds. Her Harris-Benedict equation would work out as follows:

$$BMR = 655 + (4.3 \times 190) + (4.7 \times 66) - (4.7 \times 39)$$
$$BMR = 655 + 819 + 310.2 - 183.3 = 1600.9 \text{ calories}$$

Adding Activity Level to Your BMR

Your BMR is your body's energy need for survival, but it doesn't take physical activity into account. Therefore, to get the best estimate of your daily calorie need, take your BMR and multiply it by a number based on your level of activity. For example, Nancy reports that she works at a desk job, doesn't exercise and is often too tired to do a lot of walking. So Nancy's activity level would be considered *sedentary*.

If we multiply Nancy's BMR by 1.2, which is the activity-level constant for someone who is sedentary, we find that Nancy requires 1,901.08 calories (rounded off to 1,900) a day to maintain her weight of 190 pounds. If Nancy wants to lose weight, she must reduce her daily calorie intake so that it is below 1,900 calories.

IF THIS DESCRIBES YOUR LIFESTYLE	YOU ARE CONSIDERED	MULTIPLY YOUR BMR BY
You either do not work or you work at a desk job. Your commute to work involves very little walking. You do not exercise and have no energy for more than lounging in the evening.	Sedentary	1.2
You take care of light household responsibilities and are able to do some walking.	Fairly Active	1.3
You spend some of the day on your feet or walking and you exercise for 20 to 30 minutes 2 to 3 times a week.	Moderately Active	1.5
You like to go for long walks or hikes and are always on your feet. You exercise with moderate intensity for 45 to 60 minutes 4 to 5 times a week.	Very Active	1.7

How to Reduce Your Calorie Intake to Lose Weight

In order to lose one pound of body fat, your body requires a deficit of 3,500 calories. So if you decrease your calorie intake by 500 calories a day for a week, you should lose one pound (500 x 7 = 3,500). For Nancy to lose one pound a week, she needs to reduce her calorie intake to 1,400 calories a day (1,900 − 500 = 1,400). However, if Nancy would rather make a smaller reduction in her daily calorie intake, she can still successfully lose weight. For instance, if she decreases her intake by just 300 calories a day (eating a total of 1,600 calories), she would lose a pound in about 12 days.

There are many options when deciding how many calories to reduce daily. The best recommendation I have is to start with a 500-calorie a day reduction. If you feel too hungry, add calories so you will have a net reduction of about 300 calories per day. If you begin with a 500-calorie deficit and are not losing at an acceptable rate, you may wish to decrease you calories by 700 a day.

You should explore your most pressing reasons for losing weight before deciding how much you will reduce your calories. For example, some of my patients tell me that they would prefer to reduce their calories as much as possible when they first begin their diet to get that motivating shot in the arm. On the other hand, some patients tell me that they are committed to eating healthier and making lasting lifestyle changes and are in no hurry to lose all their weight quickly. Think about these factors before deciding how many calories to cut from your daily diet.

What's Your Ideal Weight?

This is a question that may be difficult for you to answer, or you may find that your answer to this question changes over time. I always discuss weight goals with my patients on our first visit. I believe you have to know where you are going before you decide how you're going to get there. My patients often have one weight goal in mind—their lowest recorded adult weight. My suggestion is often a bit different. I base my recommendation on a patient's adult weight history and her body mass index. Your body mass index is determined by your current weight and height. It's a mathematical equation that gives you a number, or index, that correlates to relative risk of developing illnesses.

A NOTE FOR THE EXTREMELY OBESE

Some researchers believe that the Harris-Benedict Formula is not accurate for the extremely obese (see the chart on body mass index on pages 24 and 25), because it may overestimate their calorie needs. This is because extremely obese people have greater amounts of body fat and less muscle mass, and muscle requires much more energy than fat. While some researchers suggest that this group of individuals calculate the Harris-Benedict Formula using their ideal body weight instead of their actual weight, this may actually underestimate calorie needs. Researchers are looking for ways to more accurately determine calorie levels for everyone. But in the meantime, I suggest that you use your actual weight in the Harris-Benedict equation but keep in mind that this may be a bit of an overestimate. As you continue with the plan, taking note of how much you are losing a week versus how hungry you feel will give you a better idea of how many calories you should take in daily, and whether you need to make adjustments.

According to the National Institutes of Health a body mass index of between 18.5 and 24.9 is considered average. A BMI of 25 to 29.9 is considered overweight. A BMI of over 30 defines obesity: 30 to 34.9 is Class I obesity; 35 to 39.9 is Class II obesity; and any reading over 40 is considered Class III or extreme obesity. Take a look at the BMI chart on the next two pages for more information.

Body Mass Index Table

BMI	AVERAGE						OVERWEIGHT					OBESITY: CLASS I				
	19	20	21	22	23	24	25	26	27	28	29	30	31	32	33	34
Height (inches)	Body weight (pounds)															
58	91	96	100	105	110	115	119	124	129	134	138	143	148	153	158	162
59	94	99	104	109	114	119	124	128	133	138	143	148	153	158	163	168
60	97	102	107	112	118	123	128	133	138	143	148	153	158	163	168	174
61	100	106	111	116	122	127	132	137	143	148	153	158	164	169	174	180
62	104	109	115	120	126	131	136	142	147	153	158	164	169	175	180	186
63	107	113	118	124	130	135	141	146	152	158	163	169	175	180	186	191
64	110	116	122	128	134	140	145	151	157	163	169	174	180	186	192	197
65	114	120	126	132	138	144	150	156	162	168	174	180	186	192	198	204
66	118	124	130	136	142	148	155	161	167	173	179	186	192	198	204	210
67	121	127	134	140	146	153	159	166	172	178	185	191	198	204	211	217
68	125	131	138	144	151	158	164	171	177	184	190	197	203	210	216	223
69	128	135	142	149	155	162	169	176	182	189	196	203	209	216	223	230
70	132	139	146	153	160	167	174	181	188	195	202	209	216	222	229	236
71	136	143	150	157	165	172	179	186	193	200	208	215	222	229	236	243
72	140	147	154	162	169	177	184	191	199	206	213	221	228	235	242	250
73	144	151	159	166	174	182	189	197	204	212	219	227	235	242	250	257
74	148	155	163	171	179	186	194	202	210	218	225	233	241	249	256	264
75	152	160	168	176	184	192	200	208	216	224	232	240	248	256	264	272
76	156	164	172	180	189	197	205	213	221	230	238	246	254	263	271	279

INSTRUCTIONS: Find your height in the left-hand column. Move across to the number closest to your weight. The number at the top of the column is the BMI for your height and weight. Pounds have been rounded off.

Body Mass Index Table

OBESITY: CLASS II					EXTREME OBESITY: CLASS III											
35	36	37	38	39	40	41	42	43	44	45	46	47	48	49	50	BMI
Body weight (pounds)																Height (inches)
167	172	177	181	186	191	196	201	205	210	215	220	224	229	234	239	58
173	178	183	188	193	198	203	208	212	217	222	227	232	237	242	247	59
179	184	189	194	199	204	209	215	220	225	230	235	240	245	250	255	60
185	190	195	201	206	211	217	222	227	232	238	243	248	254	259	264	61
191	196	202	207	213	218	224	229	235	240	246	251	256	262	267	273	62
197	203	208	214	220	225	231	237	242	248	254	259	265	270	278	282	63
204	209	215	221	227	232	238	244	250	256	262	267	273	279	285	291	64
210	216	222	228	234	240	246	252	258	264	270	276	282	288	294	300	65
216	223	229	235	241	247	253	260	266	272	278	284	291	297	303	309	66
223	230	236	242	249	255	261	268	274	280	287	293	299	306	312	319	67
230	236	243	249	256	262	269	276	282	289	295	302	308	315	322	328	68
236	243	250	257	263	270	277	284	291	297	304	311	318	324	331	338	69
243	250	257	264	271	278	285	292	299	306	313	320	327	334	341	348	70
250	257	265	272	279	286	293	301	308	315	322	329	338	343	351	358	72
258	265	272	279	287	294	302	309	316	324	331	338	346	353	361	368	72
265	272	280	288	295	302	310	318	325	333	340	348	355	363	371	378	73
272	280	287	295	303	311	319	326	334	342	350	358	365	373	381	389	74
279	287	295	303	311	319	327	335	343	351	359	367	375	383	391	399	75
287	295	304	312	320	328	336	344	353	361	369	377	385	394	402	410	76

What's Your BMI?

The following simple equation tells you your body mass index:

$$BMI = \frac{703 \times weight\ (in\ pounds)}{height\ (in\ inches)\ squared}\ (divided\ by)$$

Let's plug in the numbers, using the formula above, for our friend Nancy.

$$Nancy's\ BMI = \frac{703 \times 190}{66 \times 66}\ (divided\ by)\ \frac{133570}{4356} = 30.663$$

While the BMI is an important and useful tool in determining a reasonable and healthy weight goal, it does have its drawbacks. The formula does not take into account gender, muscle mass or bone density. Therefore, if you are very large boned or have a higher muscle mass, your BMI may rate your health risk as higher than it really is.

The American Heart Association recommends that for best cardiac health, Americans should try to achieve a BMI of 25 or lower. That's because once your BMI exceeds 25, statistically speaking, your risk of heart disease increases. Another benchmark in evaluating your BMI is 30. Once again, there is a dramatic increase in health risk at this mark.

If your BMI is 42, it may be difficult to achieve and maintain a BMI under 25, for reasons that are often outside your control. So, you need to consider many factors while planning your ultimate weight goal. Remember that it takes a loss of only 5 to 10 percent of your total body weight to significantly improve your health. I see this all the time. Patients report a reduction in breathing difficulties, less pain in joints and increased energy with small losses of weight. Use the exercise goal sheets provided on pages 156 and 160 to guide you through the process of determining your ideal weight.

THE PLAN

NOW THAT YOU'VE DECIDED HOW MANY CALORIES TO EAT every day in order to lose weight, you need to know what to eat. This is where things get a bit easier. On page 29 are menu patterns for various calorie levels. We've also given you food lists from which to construct your diet. These food lists and how you use them in meal planning are described later in this chapter. There are 30 days of healthy menus provided in this book, as well.

The Right Stuff: Protein, Fat and Carbohydrates

There has been a tremendous amount of controversy over how these three nutrients—protein, fat and carbohydrates—should be distributed in meals for optimal health and success with weight loss. I've been in practice long enough that I can't even remember all the fad diets that have come and gone. There's the high-protein plan, the high-fat plan, the high-carbohydrate plan, as well as many other variations. But eliminating whole food groups will deprive your body of essential nutrients and rob you of the protective health benefits that these nutrients offer. The plan in this book is one that has worked for thousands of my patients, and I can say with certainty that patients following this plan are not just losing weight, but also eating for optimum health.

The Carbohydrate-Hunger Connection

In your quest to lose weight in the past, you may have tried to cut fat and calories by eating more carbohydrates, a food most women strongly crave. This may have left you hungry, craving sweets and feeling miserable—so much so that you admitted defeat and gave up your plan to lose weight. Guess what? You weren't lacking the right motivation or focus to be able to follow your weight-loss plan, you were, however, lacking the right plan for dieting success.

Why is it that eating too many carbohydrates makes you hungry and increases your food cravings? The answer has to do with a hormonal response from your body. Whenever you eat a carbohydrate-rich food (like a bagel), it is quickly digested and absorbed. This causes a quick rise in your blood sugar level, which stimulates the pancreas to secrete insulin—a hormone that transports sugar from your bloodstream across the cell membrane to provide energy and helps keep your blood sugar levels within a normal range.

When your blood sugar rises quickly, sugar in the bloodstream is transported across cell membranes with lightning speed. But since your body doesn't need all this energy at once, most of it is stored as fat. In addition, the quick transport of energy from the bloodstream to the cells causes a quick drop in blood sugar levels (called rebound hypoglycemia, or low blood sugar). It's this rebound hypoglycemia that causes increased hunger and heightened food cravings as well as fatigue and headache.

Certain types of carbohydrates raise blood sugar levels more quickly than others. The rate at which a food raises blood sugar levels is measured by its glycemic index. The higher the glycemic index, the faster that food will raise blood glucose levels. In general, sugar, white bread, bagels, white potatoes, white rice, cookies, cakes, muffins, fruit juice and refined cereals have a high glycemic index. Research shows that eating a diet abundant in high-glycemic foods results in increased insulin levels, heightened hunger and weight gain.

The *Woman's Day* weight-loss plan is based on this cutting-edge research about carbohydrates and the glycemic index. It emphasizes foods that have a low glycemic index, such as beans, bulgur wheat, pearled barley, lentils, high-fiber cereals, whole-grain bread, sweet potatoes and most vegetables. The food lists recommend choosing lower glycemic carbohydrates, and the sample daily menus and recipes stress low-glycemic eating.

Some Fat Is Good for You

We now know that fat-free or very lowfat diets do not seem to work for the majority of people trying to lose weight. We also know that small amounts of certain kinds of fats make you feel more satisfied for longer periods of time, slow down digestion and appear to have a positive effect on your cholesterol levels. Based on these and other research data, the menu patterns have been designed to provide about 25 percent of calories from fat. Recommended healthy fat choices include avocado, flaxseeds, flaxseed oil, olive oil, canola oil, nuts and olives. Flaxseeds and flaxseed oil are rich in heart-healthy omega-3 fatty acids and are believed to protect against certain forms of cancer.

Protein—In moderation

The remaining calories in this plan come from protein, which is necessary for the development of hormones and antibodies (for a strong immune system) and to build muscle mass. But unlike many of the popular "high-protein" diets of recent years, the *Woman's Day* weight-loss plan suggests a relatively moderate amount of protein, since too much can overwork kidneys, increase cholesterol levels and drain bones of calcium. In addition, the plan emphasizes lean sources of protein, such as chicken and fish.

Five Menu Patterns

The meal patterns below get less than half of their total calories from carbohydrates (with a range of 44 to 49 percent), 24 to 27 percent of total calories from fat and and 27 to 29 percent of calories from protein. Use the pattern that comes closest to your daily calorie needs minus the deficit you decided will work for you (usually 300 to 1,000 fewer calories a day).

If your calorie level for weight loss falls in between or above the suggested patterns listed, you can easily make the necessary adjustments. Use the lower calorie level as your pattern base and adjust the calorie content up by adding a serving of these food groups to total the calorie level you need:

	1,000*	1,200**	1,400	1,600	1,800
Protein servings	6	8	9	10	12
Bread/starch serving	3	4	5	6	6
Fruit servings	2	2	2	3	3
Vegetable servings	4 or more	4 or more	5 or more	6 or more	6 or more
Dairy servings	2	2	2	2	2
Fat servings	3	4	5	5	6
Actual calories	1015	1220	1410	1615	1830
Total protein (grams)	75	84	96	112	126
Total carbohydrate (grams)	119	134	154	201	201
Total fat (grams)	27	36	43	45	54

* Only reduce your calorie intake to this level if you have a very small frame and are sedentary.
** This is by far the most frequently prescribed calorie level for women, so the sample menus provided in this book are designed for this calorie level.

protein (40 calories per serving), bread/starch (80 calories per serving), fruits (60 calories per serving), vegetables (25 calories per serving), dairy (90 calories per serving) or fat (45 calories per serving).

For example, if your calorie needs total 2,050 for the day and you would like to lose about one pound a week, you should follow a plan of 1,550 calories a day. You can simply modify the 1,400-calorie plan by adding one serving of bread/starch (80 calories), one serving of protein (40 calories) and one serving of vegetables (25 calories). You can use this same strategy to increase the calories of your food pattern by 100 calories if you are too hungry or to make reductions if you feel you're losing too slowly.

HOW TO USE THE FOOD CHOICE SYSTEM IN MENU PLANNING

Food Choice Lists

Foods with similar nutrient composition and calorie content are grouped together to make menu planning and calorie counting a snap. Seven food choice groups are listed below. Refer to your calorie level menu pattern for your daily allotment in each food group. You can plan your daily meals by referring to your pattern and making your choices (and portion sizes) from the lists below.

The items listed in each group represent one serving. You can "exchange" any item for a different item on the same list of food choices. You may double or triple the serving size to create a reasonable portion size. For example, although ⅓ of a cup of wild rice is one serving of bread/starch, this is not a usual portion size. Serve yourself ⅔ of a cup of wild rice and count your portion as 2 bread/starch servings. Each list is further subdivided to give you guidance in improving the quality of your diet. Choosing most of your foods from the "best choices" category is recommended. These are the healthiest choices and generally have the lowest glycemic index.

The food choice system is a valuable tool that will provide you an infinite number of possibilities in meal planning. Refer to the lists often to become more familiar with how different foods stack up. Before you know it, you'll have most of the information ingrained in your memory. The sample menus in the book will help get you started.

PROTEINS

Each serving contains 7 grams of protein, 0–5 grams of fat and 35–55 calories.

BEST CHOICES

FOOD ITEM	SERVING SIZE
Beans, cooked (kidney, black, garbanzo, etc.)	½ cup*
Cheese, fat-free	1 oz
Chicken breast, no skin	1 oz
Cottage cheese, nonfat or 1% fat	¼ cup
Egg whites	2 whites
Egg substitute	¼ cup
Fish fillet (flounder, sole, scrod, turbot, etc.)	1 oz
Luncheon meats, reduced-fat (with about 3 g or less of fat per oz)	1 oz
Salmon, swordfish, sardines or herring	1 oz
Shellfish (clams, lobster, scallops, shrimp)	1 oz
Tofu (soybean curd)**	2 oz
Tuna, canned in water	1 oz
Turkey, breast or leg, no skin	1 oz
Vegetarian burger (2½-oz patty)	1 patty*

SECOND-BEST CHOICES

FOOD ITEM	SERVING SIZE
Beef, lean (flank steak, London broil, tenderloin or roast beef)	1 oz
Cheese, reduced-fat (with 5 g or less of fat per oz)	1 oz
Chicken, dark meat, no skin	1 oz
Frank, reduced-fat (with 1–3 g of fat and about 50 calories each)	1 each
Lamb, roast or lean chop	1 oz
Mozzarella cheese, part-skim	1 oz

* Count as 1 protein and 1 bread/starch.
** If you are pregnant or nursing or are a breast cancer survivor you should talk to your doctor before consuming any phytoestrogen-rich foods.

FOOD ITEM	SERVING SIZE
Pork, tenderloin or ham	1 oz
Veal, roast or lean chop	1 oz

FOOD ITEM	SERVING SIZE
Beef, prime cut or ground	1 oz
Cottage cheese, 4% fat	¼ cup
Egg, whole	1 each

BREAD/STARCHES

Each serving contains 3 grams of protein, 15 grams of carbohydrate and 80 calories.

BEST CHOICES

FOOD ITEM	SERVING SIZE
Barley, cooked	⅓ cup
Bread (whole-wheat, multigrain, pumpernickel or rye)	1 slice
Bread, light (whole-wheat, rye or whole-grain)	2 slices
Bulgur wheat, cooked*	½ cup
Cold cereal, high-fiber (with more than 5 g of fiber per serving)	¾ cup
English muffin, whole-wheat	½ muffin
Green peas, cooked	½ cup
Lima beans, cooked	½ cup
Oatmeal, cooked	½ cup
Pasta, whole-wheat, cooked	½ cup
Pita pocket, mini whole-wheat	1 each
Rice, wild, cooked	⅓ cup
Weave-type wheat crackers, reduced-fat (with more than 2 g of fiber per serving)	4 crackers

* Bulgur wheat is a Middle Eastern grain available at most health food stores.

SECOND-BEST CHOICES

FOOD ITEM	SERVING SIZE
Bagel (whole-wheat, pumpernickel or rye)	¼ (1 oz)
Couscous, cooked	⅓ cup
Corn, fresh or canned	½ cup
Egg noodles, cooked	½ cup
English muffin, white	½ muffin
Pasta, cooked (bow-tie, spaghetti, etc.)	½ cup
Pita pocket (regular size)	½ pita
Popcorn (hot-air popped or microwave light)	3 cups popped
Potato, sweet or yam	3 oz
Rice, brown, cooked	⅓ cup
Roll, whole-grain, medium	½ roll
Sesame flatbread (6½ by 1½ in)	2 slices
Wheat crackers, reduced-fat, small	12 each

CHOOSE INFREQUENTLY (HIGHER GLYCEMIC FOODS)

FOOD ITEM	SERVING SIZE
Bagels, white	¼ (1 oz)
Bread, white	1 slice
Bread, white, light	2 slices
Breadsticks	2 medium
Cold cereal, refined (with more than 5 g of fiber per serving)	¾ cup
Crackers, saltine type	6 crackers
Graham crackers	3 squares
Hamburger roll, white	½ roll
Potato, white	3 oz
Pretzels	3–4 oz
Rice, white	⅓ cup
Rice cakes, all varieties	2 large

FRUITS

Each serving contains 15 grams of carbohydrate and 60 calories.

BEST CHOICES

FOOD ITEM	SERVING SIZE
Apple, pear, peach, plum or nectarine, with skin	1 medium
Cherries, fresh	12 each
Dried apricots	7 halves
Grapefruit, fresh	½
Melon cubes, cantaloupe or honeydew	1 cup
Strawberries, blackberries, raspberries, blueberries	1 cup

SECOND-BEST CHOICES

FOOD ITEM	SERVING SIZE
Banana	1 small
Clementine	2 each
Canned fruit, packed in unsweetened juice	½ cup
Grapes, fresh	15 each
Orange	1 medium
Tangerine	1 large

CHOOSE INFREQUENTLY (HIGHER GLYCEMIC FOODS)

FOOD ITEM	SERVING SIZE
Juice (orange, apple, etc., unsweetened)	½ cup
Juice (prune or cranberry)	⅓ cup
Juice, reduced-sugar cranberry	1 cup
Dried prunes	3 whole
Kiwi	1 whole
Pineapple, fresh or canned	¾ cup cubed
Raisins	2 Tbsp
Watermelon	1¼ cup cubed

VEGETABLES

Each serving contains 5 grams of carbohydrate and 25 calories.

BEST CHOICES

FOOD ITEM	SERVING SIZE
Vegetables, steamed or microwave-cooked (cauliflower, broccoli, spinach, etc.)	½ cup
Grilled vegetables*	½ cup
Raw vegetables (broccoli florets, celery, cucumber sticks and zucchini strips)	1 cup
Raw salad greens	1 cup

SECOND-BEST CHOICES

FOOD ITEM	SERVING SIZE
Canned vegetables, any variety	½ cup
Marinara sauce	⅓ cup
Tomato juice	4 oz
Vegetable juice, regular or low-sodium	4 oz

CHOOSE INFREQUENTLY (HIGHER GLYCEMIC FOODS)

FOOD ITEM	SERVING SIZE
Beets, cooked	½ cup

LOWFAT DAIRY

Each serving contains approximately 8 grams of protein, 0–4 grams of fat, 12 grams of carbohydrate and 80–120 calories.

BEST CHOICES

FOOD ITEM	SERVING SIZE
Milk, nonfat, skim-plus** or 1% lowfat	8 oz
Yogurt, nonfat, plain or artificially sweetened	8 oz

*   Grill using nonstick cooking spray.
** Skim-plus is skim milk with added calcium.

FOOD ITEM	SERVING SIZE
Milk, 2% reduced-fat	8 oz
Pudding, flavored, sugar-free, fat-free*	½ cup
Yogurt, lowfat plain	8 oz

CHOOSE INFREQUENTLY (FOODS HIGHER IN FAT/SUGAR)

FOOD ITEM	SERVING SIZE
Milk, whole	6 oz
Yogurt, lowfat flavored (vanilla, coffee or lemon)	4 oz

FATS

Each serving contains 5 grams of fat and 45 calories.

BEST CHOICES

FOOD ITEM	SERVING SIZE
Almonds	6 whole
Avocado	⅛ medium
Olives, black	8 large
Flaxseeds, ground**, †	1 Tbsp
Flaxseed oil†, ††	1 tsp
Margarine, reduced-fat, trans-fatty-acid free	1 Tbsp
Olives, green stuffed	10 small
Oil (canola or olive)	1 tsp
Peanuts	10 small
Peanut butter, natural	2 tsp
Salad dressing, oil-and-vinegar base	1 Tbsp
Sunflower seeds	1 Tbsp
Walnuts	4 halves

*   Available as a mix at your grocery store.
** Find in health food stores. Rich in omega-3 fatty acids. Store in refrigerator and grind before using.
†   If you are pregnant or nursing or are a breast cancer survivor you should talk to your doctor before consuming any phytoestrogen-rich food.
†† Do not use flaxseed oil in cooking as it is heat sensitive. Use on salads and cooked vegetables.

FOOD ITEM	SERVING SIZE
Bacon, Canadian	1 slice
Cashews	6 whole
Cream cheese, light	1½ Tbsp
Oil, sunflower, corn, safflower	1 tsp
Margarine, reduced-fat	1 Tbsp
Mayonnaise, light	1 Tbsp
Peanut butter, creamy or chunky	2 tsp

CHOOSE INFREQUENTLY (FOODS HIGH IN SATURATED FAT)

FOOD ITEM	SERVING SIZE
Bacon, pork	1 slice
Butter	1 tsp
Cream cheese	1 Tbsp
Margarine, stick	1 tsp
Mayonnaise	1 tsp
Sausage	1 link (½ oz)
Sour cream	1 tsp

MISCELLANEOUS FOOD CHOICES
(FOR OCCASIONAL INDULGENCES)

The following food items can be occasionally substituted for a serving of bread/starch. Each serving contains about 80–110 calories.

FOOD ITEM	SERVING SIZE
Beer, lite	12 oz
Beer, nonalcoholic	12 oz
Champagne, dry	4 oz
Cheese, full fat	1 oz
Chocolate pieces (size of Hershey's Kisses)	3 small
Cookies, chocolate chip (2½ inch in diameter)	2 each
Cookies, fig bars	2 each

FOOD ITEM	SERVING SIZE
Frozen yogurt, reduced-fat	½ cup
Potato chips	10 each
Soda, regular	8 oz
Tortilla chips, baked	10 large
Wine, dry, white or red	4 oz

Note: Food choice lists are based on the food exchange system from the American Dietetic Association and the American Diabetes Association.

Ten Freebies for Guilt-Free Eating

RAW VEGETABLES Keep celery sticks, cucumber strips, broccoli florets, etc., in the fridge. Use salsa, plain nonfat yogurt or fat-free dressing as a dip.

FAT-FREE, SUGAR-FREE HOT CHOCOLATE One cup a day.

SUGAR-FREE GELATIN Up to two servings daily. Top with up to 2 table-spoons of fat-free nondairy whipped topping.

SUGAR-FREE ICE POPS With 10 calories or fewer per pop. Have up to two ice pops a day.

BEVERAGES Diet soda, sugar-free fruit juices, sugar-free flavored iced teas, herbal teas, coffee or tea. No limit on daily amounts. However, you should limit caffeinated beverages, such as diet colas, coffee and tea, to no more than three servings a day, because caffeine increases stomach acid, which can make you hungry. There is no need to measure the milk you put in your coffee or tea.

VINEGARS Wine, cider, rice, balsamic or flavored. Use to add flavor to salads and as marinades for meats.

SALSA Can really spice up your food. Add to meats, or use as a sauce for steamed vegetables. Since salsa is high in sodium, limit the amount you use if you need to restrict your sodium intake.

PICKLES Add to a sandwich or eat plain to add crunch to your lunch. One whole pickle has only 10 calories, but keep in mind that they are also high in sodium.

PLAIN BOUILLON SOUP You can have one to two cups a day. Choose the unsalted version if you need to restrict your sodium intake.

FRESH HERBS AND SPICES Make a plain broiled chicken much more interesting. Add fresh dill, parsley and oregano to your foods during meal preparation.

A Note for Diabetics

This plan is acceptable for many diabetics, but you must first get clearance from your doctor before starting this or any weight-loss program. Your doctor needs to be informed about changes in your diet and physical activity, since certain medications may need to be adjusted if you're cutting calories and losing weight. Also, be sure to discuss the protein level in this plan with your doctor and/or dietitian, since the menu plans in this book may have too much protein for diabetics who have a reduction in kidney function.

Type 1 diabetics who are on insulin injections need to discuss carefully with a physician, dietitian or certified diabetes specialist how to adjust insulin dosage while following a reduced-calorie plan. Both Type 1 and Type 2 diabetics should increase the frequency of daily blood sugar testing while losing weight and making changes in medication type or dosages. Don't forget to be prepared to treat unexpected hypoglycemia. Carry glucose tablets or readily available sugar sources for a quick remedy for hypoglycemia.

The American Diabetes Association reports that if your blood sugars are in good control, you can eat up to 10 percent of your total calories as sugar. Once again, check with your doctor or dietitian to see if you rate as a diabetic in good control. If you prefer, you can substitute artificially sweetened cookies for regular cookies on the menus, or use a sugar substitute in any of the recipes that list sugar as an ingredient.

A Note for People with Hypertension

People with high blood pressure can follow this plan, too, but it is essential that you first speak with your doctor. If you are taking medicine to help lower your blood pressure, you will need to talk with your doctor about how weight loss might interact with this medication. Your doctor may want to monitor your blood pressure more frequently and adjust your medication as you lose weight.

Continue to reduce the sodium in your diet as prescribed by your doctor or dietitian. If you wish, you can substitute the items on the daily menus that have a higher sodium content (such as ham, ready-to-use canned soups and cheese) with low-sodium alternatives. If you have any concerns, speak with your doctor and/or dietitian for individualized guidance. There is information in the Resources section (page 163) on how to find a registered dietitian in your area.

A Note for Vegetarians

A vegetarian diet is a healthy and wise choice, but even healthy foods eaten in excess can help you pile on the pounds. I've made a list on page 41 of some typical vegetarian foods and how you can count them in your daily menu patterns. Some of the vegetarian food items you choose may vary slightly depending upon different manufacturers, but this list will give you a good idea of how to count some of the most common vegetarian food choices. Refer to the nutrition labels for guidance on foods not on the list. Other vegetarian foods, such as beans, rice and bulgur wheat, can be found on the general food lists.

A Note for Lactose-Intolerant People

The menu patterns in this book include the recommended amounts of calcium-rich dairy foods, which you may be unable to eat. However, many of my patients use lactose-reduced or lactose-free milk and milk products. Soy milk and soy cheese are other options for you to consider. (Values for soy milk and soy cheese can be found on page 41.)

FOOD	AMOUNT	CALORIES	COUNT AS
Soy milk, plain	8 oz	110	1 dairy
Soy milk, flavored	8 oz	140	1 dairy, ½ fruit
Soy cheese, fat-free	1 oz	35	1 protein
Soy breakfast link	1-oz link	50	1 protein
Meatless salami	3 slices/2 oz	130	1 protein, 1 fat
Veggie dog	1 link	80	1 protein, ½ bread/starch
Veggie burger	2½-oz patty	120	1 protein, 1 bread/starch
Veggie bacon	3 slices/2 oz	80	2 proteins
Soy chicken nuggets	4 nuggets/3 oz	160	1 bread/starch, 2 proteins
Tofu, extra-firm	4 oz	100	1½ proteins, ½ fat
Tofu ravioli	3½ oz or 1 cup	180	2 bread/starches, 1 protein
Soy tempeh	3 oz	150	1 bread/starch, 2 proteins
Vegetarian Chili*	1½-cup serving	325	3 bread/starches, 2 vegetables, 1 protein

*Recipe, page 137

Getting Started Checklist

Be sure to check off the following before starting your new diet:

_____ I checked with my doctor before starting this program.

_____ I will take a daily multivitamin/mineral supplement.

_____ I will take a calcium supplement if I can't take in all the calcium-rich foods on the menu plan (see Chapter 3 for calcium needs and a list of the calcium content of various foods).

_____ I will complete the goal worksheets provided in this book.

_____ I will keep a daily food journal.

_____ I will stock my kitchen with recommended food before I begin the program.

_____ I will seek support from my friends and family.

What You Should Expect in Terms of Weight Loss

Most of my patients are very interested in knowing how fast, or at what rate, they can expect to lose. The rate at which people lose weight varies greatly. You can expect to lose the greatest amount of weight in the first month or two of dieting. I've seen patients lose as much as four to five pounds a week and as little as half a pound a week. What's really important is that you continue to make progress.

It's also important to note that, over time, even small losses in weight add up to a significant total loss. Use the weight-loss graph on page 159 to help you evaluate your progress over a period of time. The following are variables that may affect your rate of weight loss:

- How much total weight you have to lose. The more you have to lose, the greater your rate of weight loss will be.

- Your past weight-loss history. If you've dieted before, you know from past experience whether your weight just falls right off or appears to be held onto your body with Krazy Glue. Your own genetic makeup and metabolism controls this to some degree.

- How active you can be. It you have physical limits on what you can do to exercise, this will impact your weight loss. I have patients who are disabled who can successfully lose weight, but they need to accept a slower rate of weight loss.

- The length of time you are dieting. Some of my patients experience a slowdown in weight loss—the dreaded plateau—while following the program. Sometimes, fluid weight gain can affect your reading on the scale, and it can appear as if you haven't lost any body fat over the week. Women are more prone to this, as fluid shifts occur with changes in monthly hormonal levels. This situation can be very discouraging when you've done everything right, and you don't get the result you expect. If this happens, try to keep a level head and don't get discouraged. Stay on your plan. Avoid cutting calories lower or overexercising to remedy the situation. Sometimes, letting time pass is the best remedy. The best advice I can give to you about evaluating your rate of weight loss is to be realistic, don't get easily discouraged and never, never, never give up!

PART TWO

Losing Weight During Each Stage of the Everchanging Female Life Cycle

3. The Early Years

YOU JUST DON'T GET IT. You have youth on your side, you eat somewhat healthily, you're fairly active, and yet you're overweight. Meanwhile, your size-two buddy eats junk food all the time, sits around most of the day reading and wouldn't know how to step on a treadmill, let alone what to do with a set of hand weights. But try not to waste your time and energy bemoaning how unfair and arbitrary your body's metabolism is. Instead, put all that energy into something positive—taking charge and making the changes necessary to achieve your goal of losing weight.

The truth is that you aren't necessarily what you eat. Most of the overweight young women I counsel eat much healthier than their average-weight peers. Don't get me wrong, these women need to make changes, but it's still surprising to me that their bodies will maintain such a high body weight without obvious cause. Genetics undoubtedly plays a role in an unhealthy, higher body weight. You may not be able to control your genetics (at least not yet), but you can control your environment.

YOUNG WOMEN

"THE FRESHMAN 15." My college-bound patients who have a tendency toward weight gain nearly hyperventilate upon hearing this frightening phrase, which refers to the folk wisdom that college freshmen will gain 15 pounds of body weight along with all that knowledge. The college years are challenging for the student trying either to lose weight or maintain a healthy weight.

Another group of patients—single working women—tell me their active social lives interfere with their ability to cut calories. Newlyweds tell me that ever since they returned home from their honeymoon, they've been gaining weight in leaps and bounds. Many smart women see me for pre-conception weight-loss counseling. They know that achieving a healthy weight before getting pregnant is good for them and their baby-to-be.

There's good news for all women in early adulthood. First, the healthy habits you create now can last you a lifetime. The rest of the story is that with some planning, all the challenges that you face can be met and conquered.

THE COLLEGE YEARS

THE JURY IS STILL OUT on whether the "Freshman 15" is fact or fiction, so don't let the phrase send a chill down your spine. However, the truth is that special circumstances during the college years make it easy to lose sight of your plans to eat right and exercise. Late-night snacking while studying, limited choices at the school cafeteria and an erratic schedule set the stage for weight gain and lack of exercise.

In a novel approach to help college freshmen avoid weight gain, researchers at Iowa State University observed the effect that taking a nutrition course had on weight gain in freshmen. They followed 40 female college students for 16 months and found that those who took a college-level nutrition course lost a small amount of weight over the study period. However, those in the control group who didn't attend a nutrition course gained weight.

Increased levels of stress also play a role in discouraging college students from eating right. My patients tell me that there are many reasons they feel stressed during their college years. It's an exciting time, but also one filled with anticipation and decision-making. It's a time when you worry about the choices you make and how those decisions will affect your future. With all this on your mind, getting to the gym is not likely to be a priority. Ironically, eating right and exercising will enable you to make your choices and feel better about yourself and your future. Many of my college patients tell me that taking charge of their lives by eating healthily and exercising gives them the energy they need to face all the other challenges of the day.

Late-night snacking is a major contributor to college weight gain. Staying up late to study for an exam or to finish that term paper will automatically demand that you consume additional calories. If you go to bed at a reasonable hour, you sleep through your hunger pangs. On nights when you're cramming for a test, though, you'll undoubtedly act on those pangs. If you're studying with a group, it's a safe bet that someone will order Chinese food or a pizza or will start ripping open an enormous bag of chips. Don't let yourself get sucked into eating these high-fat, high-calorie snack foods. Have a better plan for snacking in the wee hours of the morning. Take a look at some healthier, lower calorie alternatives. It may take a bit more time and effort to have healthier snacks ready, but your shrinking waistline will thank you.

College students who live at home or have access to a full kitchen will

Snack Alternatives for College Days

INSTEAD OF	CHOOSE	SAVE (CALORIES)
2 slices pizzeria-style pizza	English Muffin Pizza: 1 whole-wheat English muffin topped with tomato sauce and 1 oz part-skim mozzarella cheese	500
2 oz potato chips	1 oz pretzel sticks dipped in 1 Tbsp peanut butter	100
A plate of cheesy nachos	10 large baked tortilla chips with salsa	260
1 oz mixed nuts	3 cups microwave light popcorn	90
1 pt premium ice cream	1 no-sugar-added, chocolate-dipped ice cream bar	450
Half a 9-oz box small reduced-fat wheat crackers	7 weave-type, reduced-fat crackers and 1 oz reduced-fat Cheddar cheese	350
1 oz gummy bears and 2 oz licorice	A protein bar*	170
	TOTAL CALORIES SAVED	1920

*Refer to the "Eating Healthy on the Run" section of this chapter for tips on choosing the right protein bar.

have fewer obstacles to eating healthy snack alternatives (see Snack Alternatives for College Days, *left*). Don't worry if you can't use some of the suggestions because you lack some kitchen equipment. Some foods, like pretzels with peanut butter, require no refrigeration. Popcorn can be prepared in the microwave, or you can purchase a hot-air popper. A toaster is all you need to make English Muffin Pizza.

GET MOVING

EXERCISE IS ESSENTIAL TO LOSING WEIGHT and to successfully maintaining weight loss. Most of my college student patients tell me that they sleep late on days they don't have early classes and stay up late many evenings. Lack of structure in your schedule can interrupt your plans to get moving. Make exercise a top priority and plan out exercise time as soon as you get your class schedule for the semester.

Exercise Tips for College Students

SCHEDULE SPECIFIC TIME TO EXERCISE. Record those times in your daily planner along with your classes. Put as much importance on your exercise time as you would a scheduled class.

TAKE ADVANTAGE OF CAMPUS SERVICES AND BENEFITS. Most schools have a campus gym. Find out the days and times you're allowed to use the facilities and plan your workouts accordingly.

SIGN UP FOR A PHYSICAL EDUCATION CLASS. Many colleges offer tennis, golf, swimming or cross-country skiing classes. They're a great way to earn college credits, have fun and stay fit.

EQUIP YOUR ROOM WITH WHAT YOU NEED. For days when you can't get to the gym, keep a jump rope, exercise bands or free weights in your room to work out at your convenience.

> ### EATING SMART
>
> Hamburgers, hot dogs, French fries, soda, bagels, muffins and a limited salad bar: does this sound like the meal plan from Weight-Gain University? You'll have to work hard at finding the right food at school, and not just weight loss, but for health and disease protection, as well. That's right, what you eat now will affect your risk of developing diseases later in life—in your 40s and 50s and beyond.

Calcium: The Mineral That Matters

Women are notorious for skipping calcium-rich foods. They're also notorious for developing osteoporosis—about six times as often as men. Recent reports estimate that there are 20 million women in the U.S. with this brittle bone disease. Half of all women over the age of 50 have osteoporosis. You can dramatically reduce your odds of developing this disease by meeting your calcium needs now. Bone mass continues to grow in density until you're about 25, so if you've just started college, you have about seven more years to build up the strength of your bones. From about age 26 on, meeting daily calcium needs will replace daily mineral bone losses, but won't contribute to the mass of your bones. According to the new dietary reference intakes, women aged 19 to 50 need 1,000 mg of calcium daily, and women over 50 need 1,200 mg. The average woman gets 600 mg of calcium a day, 40 percent less than her body needs.

Passing up daily servings of milk and yogurt isn't the only reason women have a substantially higher incidence of osteoporosis. The other factors associated with an increased risk of developing osteoporosis are a family history of the disease, smoking, small bone structure, excessive alcohol intake or any illness that interferes with the absorption of calcium (such as Crohn's or celiac disease). Inactivity also contributes to osteoporosis. Exercise helps slow down the rate of bone loss that occurs. So meeting your calcium needs, exercising regularly and not smoking are three actions you can take now to derail osteoporosis.

Getting sufficient calcium in your diet will help you lose weight, too. Recent studies show that dieters who met their calcium needs through calcium-rich foods lost more weight than dieters who followed the same calorie-restricted diet but didn't get enough calcium. The increased weight loss in the group that ate a calcium-rich diet was substantial: They lost twice as much weight as those on a low-calorie, low-calcium diet. It seems that calcium in your body communicates with fat cells in a complicated sequence of hormonal signals that tells fat cells to stop growing.

Drinking milk on Mondays, Wednesdays and Fridays won't do the job. You need to meet your calcium requirements every day. Be sure to talk to your doctor if you can't meet your calcium needs or if you have one of the conditions that puts you at high risk for osteoporosis. Find out what you can do now to build the strongest foundation possible for the future.

Review the chart below on calcium-rich foods. It's best to get most of your calcium from the food you eat, but if you can't meet your needs through diet alone, consider taking a supplement. There are many calcium supplements on the market to choose from, but calcium citrate and calcium carbonate are the most recommended sources. Calcium citrate is often recommended because it's easily absorbed and provides a substantial amount of elemental (usable) calcium, 21 percent. Calcium carbonate con-

FOOD	AMOUNT	CALCIUM CONTENT (MG)	CALORIES
Milk, 1% lowfat	8 oz	300	120
Milk, nonfat	8 oz	300	90
Milk, nonfat, lactose-free	8 oz	300	90
Milk, soy, lowfat, calcium-fortified, plain	8 oz	300	110
Yogurt, nonfat plain	8 oz	400	90
Yogurt, artificially sweetened	8 oz	400	120
Yogurt, nonfat fruit-on-the-bottom	8 oz	400	250
Cheddar cheese, full-fat	1 oz	200	100
Cheddar cheese, reduced-fat	1 oz	200	70
Mozzarella cheese, part-skim	1 oz	200	70
Soy cheese, calcium-fortified	1 oz	200	35
Cheese, fat-free	1 oz	200	35
Orange juice, calcium-fortified	8 oz	300	120
Canned salmon, with bones	3 oz	130	200
Sardines, canned in soybean oil	4 sardines	100	180
Tofu, firm	½ cup	180	260
Spinach, boiled*	½ cup	25	120

*The absorption of calcium from vegetables is impaired by fiber.

tains even more elemental calcium, 40 percent, but requires more stomach acid for absorption, so it needs to be taken with food. Avoid overdosing on calcium. Taking more than 2,500 mg of calcium a day (from food and supplements combined or supplements alone) can cause constipation and kidney stone formation and can decrease the absorption of zinc, iron and other essential minerals your body needs.

Your physician or a dietitian are the best people to help you select the right supplement. Keep in mind that your body can absorb only about 500 mg of calcium at one time, so don't pop 1,000 mg of calcium all at once. Trying to cram all your calcium into one meal won't work either, so space milk and yogurt servings throughout the day. You can see from the list of calcium-rich foods on page 51 that making sure you get enough calcium in your diet doesn't have to wreak havoc with your weight-loss plans. One cup of nonfat milk, 8 oz of artificially sweetened yogurt and 2 oz of fat-free cheese provide 900 mg of calcium, yet total only 245 calories.

Mealtime Menu Makeover

Many of my patients who are college students make the same menu mistakes day in and day out. Take a look at the menu makeover on page 53 to see how easy it is to make healthier choices at mealtime. Not only will you cut fat and calories, you'll also increase your intake of calcium-rich foods.

When Dieting Gets Out of Control

Although it's essential to make the right food and exercise choices while you're in college, be certain that you have the full picture of your plan in clear focus. Many young women are under tremendous pressure to maintain a svelte figure. A lot of that pressure comes from within, but outside influences can affect how you feel about your body and your weight. Ignore sources that send the negative, detrimental message that it's best to achieve a "skinny" figure, and don't lose sight of your goal to achieve a "healthy" shape. Some women lose a sense of their true body image. They look at their average-size body in the mirror and see obesity where none exists.

If you have a distorted image of your body, you may be driven to cut out too many calories and to overexercise. These actions indicate that you may be

Food Mistakes College Students Make & How to Fix Them

MEAL	TYPICAL COLLEGE CHOICE	CALORIES	CALCIUM (MG)	SUGGESTED MEAL	CALORIES	CALCIUM (MG)
Breakfast	Bagel with cream cheese	500	20	⅔ cup bran-flake cereal with 1% lowfat milk and 1 cup berries	195	175
Lunch	Hamburger on a bun and French fries	950	75	Turkey sandwich on pumpernickel with lettuce & tomato, 1 tsp mayonnaise	355	65
	12 oz soda	150	0	8 oz nonfat milk	90	300
Snack	Blueberry muffin	310	35	Mocha Float*	210	350
Dinner	Large plate of pasta (3 cups) with marinara sauce	530	40	Grilled chicken breast (4 oz)	140	26
				1 cup steamed mixed vegetables	50	25
				½ baked potato (preferably a sweet potato)	80	16
				1 small salad with 1 Tbsp dressing	25 45	10 0
	12 oz lemonade	150	0	8 oz nonfat milk	90	300
Snack	2 oz potato chips	300	15	1 cup raw vegetable strips with 2 Tbsp hummus**	25 50	20 15
TOTALS		2,890	185		1,355	1,302

* See recipe section, page 146.

** Homemade (see recipe section, page 134) or ready-to-use from grocery store.

suffering from an eating disorder, such as anorexia nervosa or bulimia. Anorexia nervosa is a serious condition that requires intervention by medical doctors, therapists, nutritionists and family counselors. Anorexia can lead to malnutrition, loss of menstrual periods, infertility, early-onset osteoporosis, heart disease and even death.

Bulimia is another eating disorder that can interfere with a young woman's goal of achieving ideal health. Bulimics typically binge (overeat) and purge (intentionally vomit) food. Bulimia can lead to deterioration of the teeth, ulcers on the esophagus (the tube leading from your mouth to your stomach), kidney disease and coma. If you suspect you might be suffering from either eating disorder, please tell your doctor or family who can get you the help you need. Specific direction for anorexics and bulimics is beyond the scope of this book. You can, however, refer to the Resources section (page 163) for a list of organizations that can help you. There are many places to turn to for help. Remember, you want to achieve good health, not just weight loss.

THE SINGLE WORKING WOMAN

THE SINGLE WOMEN I COUNSEL describe social calendars filled with late nights out on weekends, drinks after work during Happy Hour and long weekends away with friends. It's a great life! However, with all that socializing comes added calories. Your social life need not suffer when you change to a healthier, lower calorie diet, but minor adjustments are in order. Juggling a hectic personal life along with a new and demanding career can put your plans for eating healthy and exercising on the back burner. Don't let it happen to you. Structure time for exercise and stick to your plan. Socialize with friends while you exercise at the gym. Go for a long walk during your lunch break and work off those Happy Hour calories. Plan your meals and snacks in advance and don't leave your daily food choices to chance.

Navigating Happy Hour

It's easy to drink lots of calories while spending time at a bar with friends. Just how many calories? Look at the chart, *right*, to compare the calorie content of various alcoholic beverages. It's pretty easy to drink 600 calories in an evening, and that's beside the extra food you'll probably be eating. Just two gin and tonics and two glasses of wine will put you at the 600-calorie mark. Drink that much alcohol three evenings a week, and in just two short weeks you'll add a whole pound to your weight. Alcohol may help relax you, but it also makes you hungrier and less focused on your plan. After a few drinks, your strategy to stick to the vegetable platter takes a hike. Instead, you find yourself diving into the fatty fried mozzarella sticks and spicy chicken wings.

ALCOHOLIC DRINK	AMOUNT	CALORIES
Nonalcoholic beer	12 oz	70
Sweet dessert wine	2 oz	90
1 shot hard liquor	1½ oz	100
Champagne	4 oz	100
Light beer	12 oz	110
Wine, red or white (dry)	6 oz	120
Gin and tonic	8 oz	180
Whiskey sour	4 oz	180
Martini	5 oz	300
Liqueur (coffee with cream)	3 oz	300
Eggnog with 2 oz rum	6 oz	300
Liqueur (53 proof)	3 oz	350
Piña colada	7 oz	400

It's best to go out with friends with a very specific plan in mind. You may decide to be the designated driver and to not drink at all. Of course, if you do decide to drink, never get behind the wheel of a car. Here are a few tips to cut down on the calories you usually consume from alcohol.

- Cut down on the time spent in the diet-challenging environment of alcohol. Arrive fashionably late.

- Try a nonalcoholic beer or tomato juice with a lime wedge.
  (Only you and the bartender will know the drink is nonalcoholic.)

- Have a nonalcoholic beverage between each alcoholic drink. For instance, have a glass of wine, a diet soda and then another glass of wine.

- Order wine spritzers of half wine and half seltzer water, or light beer.

Dieting Despite Your Significant Other

Another challenge women face is a significant other with a hearty appetite and a desire for an eating buddy. This situation can be challenging for married women, as well. However, when you're dating, the situation is a bit trickier to navigate than when you've known someone for years.

The truth is, you need all the help you can get while trying to lose weight and while maintaining your new, lower body weight. Don't let your significant other become your diet saboteur. Instead, plan ahead so the situation is kept under control. First of all, you're eating a normal healthy diet. This is not a plan that will raise eyebrows or bring a lot of attention to the fact that you're dieting. Consider using some of the following strategies to combat obstacles with your significant other.

POTENTIAL OBSTACLE	SUGGESTED ACTION
You don't want any attention placed on your new menu plan.	Respond to queries about new eating habits with a comment that you're eating healthier.
Your significant other orders 3 courses when you dine out—appetizer, entrée and dessert. You feel you should do the same.	Order 3 if you wish, but for an appetizer, have melon, vegetable soup or shrimp cocktail. For dessert have fresh berries, a scoop of ice cream or sorbet.
You want to cook your special someone a healthy meal at home, but he's big on having a large potato side dish.	Prepare the same meal for both of you, but toss some frozen French fries in the oven or microwave a baked potato for your honey.
Your significant other insists you try a bite of his decadent dessert. You know that one bite might challenge your self-control.	If your repeated refusals are ignored, be firm. Tell your partner you need support, not conflict, in your plan to eat healthier.

Eating Healthy on the Run

We live in a fast-paced world. So many tasks are performed at record speed, including eating on the run. The kind of foods that are quick and available are not usually your best choices. Use the following list to give you some on-the-run food options that are diet-friendly.

MEAL/SNACK	CHOOSE	COUNT AS	CALORIES
Breakfast	Breakfast Smoothie*	1 dairy, 1 fat, 1 fruit	200
	½ cup 1% cottage cheese, 1 cup melon cubes	2 proteins, 1 fruit	150
	2 slices multigrain bread, toasted, 2 oz reduced-fat Swiss cheese	2 bread/starches, 2 proteins	260
Lunch or Dinner	1 cup bean soup topped with 1 oz shredded reduced-fat cheese, 2 medium breadsticks, 1 apple	2 bread/starches, 2 proteins, 1 fruit	310
	8 oz nonfat plain or artificially sweetened yogurt, 4 slices whole-wheat melba toast, 1 oz part-skim mozzarella cheese, 1 pear	1 dairy, 1 bread/starch, 1 protein, 1 fruit	320
	½ cup canned kidney beans, drained and rinsed. Sauté ½ cup chopped onion and 2 garlic cloves in 1 tsp oil. Add kidney beans and heat. Serve over ⅔ cup of brown or wild rice. 1 green salad, 1 Tbsp vinaigrette dressing	1 protein, 3 bread/starches, 2 fats, 1 vegetable	405
	3 oz water-packed or vacuum-sealed tuna, 2 high-fiber crackers, 1 green salad with 1 Tbsp vinaigrette dressing	3 proteins, 1 bread/starch, 1 fat, 1 vegetable	255
	4 oz rotisserie chicken breast (no skin), 1 cup steamed vegetables, 1 small roll, 1 tsp butter	4 proteins, 2 vegetables, 2 bread/starches, 1 fat	465
Snack	Protein bar (see next page)	2 proteins, 1 bread/starch	160

*See recipe section, page 132.

Protein Bars

It's impossible to keep up with all the new protein or energy bars popping up in supermarkets, drugstores and health-food stores. Reading the labels and trying to figure out which to buy can make any dieter dizzy. But Americans have embraced this vending machine alternative for snack time, and some are nutritionally acceptable.

It's hard to make a general statement about all energy/protein bars. Clearly some are way too high in carbohydrates and calories to be helpful to dieters. I also find it problematic that these bars, which have been created to help people eat healthier, contain hydrogenated fats. Hydrogenated fats are like saturated fats and are not heart-healthy. However, some bars are low enough in calories and carbohydrates to be acceptable snacks. Many of my patients find them helpful when there's nothing appropriate to eat.

So what makes a protein bar acceptable? The mix of fat, carbohydrate, protein, total calories and fiber content are all important when evaluating a protein bar's worth. Use the following guide to help you choose a bar that will work for you.

Read the label on the bar and look for the following	
Calories	No more than 150–200 calories for the entire bar
Protein	At least 12 g
Fat	No more than 5 g (This is about 1 tsp of added fat.)
Carbohydrate	No more than 15 g
Sugar	No more than 10 g of added sugar (This is about 2 ½ tsp.)
Fiber	Look for at least 2 g. Some bars contain none at all.
Taste	Of course, it's essential that you find a protein bar that has an acceptable taste for you.

THE NEWLYWED

MANY NEWLY MARRIED WOMEN come to my office telling how they got down to their lowest weight ever for their wedding day, only to start an out-of-control eating pattern once they returned home from the honeymoon. Some women are worried about getting pregnant at their higher, unhealthy weight. Others are just plain fed up with their weight and eating habits and want to feel in control again with food.

The relief after the wedding is over and all the changes life brings to the newlywed set the stage for weight gain. This is a great time, however, to turn things around. Start your marriage and new life off with a focus on health.

Restaurant Dining Suggestions

Most newlyweds report that they eat many meals out in restaurants. They know they can save calories and money if they cook more meals at home, but this is a time in their life when they have the freedom and the desire to eat out. Don't let restaurant dining throw a monkey wrench into your plans to lose weight. Set yourself up for the best possible conditions by using the following tips.

BEFORE DINING OUT...

- Plan to dine at a restaurant you're familiar with. If you know the menu, you'll be better prepared and will have more control at mealtime. If you're joining friends and didn't choose the restaurant, call ahead to review the menu over the phone. Be sure to ask if sauces and dressings can be placed on the side for you on request.

- Decide how many calories (or daily servings of food) you are going to allot yourself. Put it all down on paper. Just like your monthly budget for money, you need to plan a budget for this meal. If you want more calories for the meal, bank some by adding an extra round of exercise before you dine out.

- Plan on a healthy snack before you leave for the restaurant. Arriving starving is a recipe for disaster. If you're going to be able to stick with your plan for less food and smaller portion sizes, you'll need to avoid heavy-duty hunger when you walk through the restaurant doors.

AT THE RESTAURANT...

- Avoid temptation: Limit or nix alcohol, and have the breadbasket removed from the table. It's easy to consume 600 calories of wine and buttered bread before your meal even arrives. If you need to munch while others are digging into the breadbasket, order your salad immediately.

- If you're having a special meal out (a birthday, for example), and you want to have dessert, try sharing one. Most restaurant serving sizes of cake have 350–600 calories. You can indulge without guilt if you're eating only half a piece.

- Enjoy your surroundings. Focus on all the reasons why dining out is special, and avoid placing all the emphasis on the meal.

AFTER THE MEAL...

- Evaluate how the evening went. Did it go as smoothly as you'd planned? Or was it a disaster because you didn't get to eat most of the day, and as soon as the aromas hit you, your plan evaporated? Either way, you need to find out what went wrong and use that information the next time you dine out.

- Get right back on track the next day. You may be hungrier the day after a special meal. This is because your body makes extra insulin in response to more carbohydrate calories eaten, which, in turn, makes you hungry. If you're hungry the day after your special meal, eat lots of vegetables. You can also add an extra ounce or two of protein at mealtime if you need to.

- Feel bloated? Go for a walk or engage in some other form of exercise. This will help burn added calories and aid in getting rid of the added fluid your body retains from the higher than usual salt intake typical of restaurant dining. Don't get on the scale for two to three days after a restaurant meal. You'll be weighing water gain, not fat gain.

Romantic Low-Calorie Dinners

Are restaurant meals cutting into your calorie and financial budgets? Some restaurant meals can easily meet or exceed an entire day's calorie allotment of 1,200 to 2,200 calories. Cook a romantic meal at home instead of going out to dinner. Set the table with candles, the good china, silver and linens. A special meal doesn't have to contain lots of fat and calories. Here are some good examples of special dinners that won't throw you off your plan to eat less fat and fewer calories.

ROMANTIC MENU #1

Salad with Tangy Vinaigrette Dressing*
Broiled Salmon with Olive Salsa*
Wild Rice with Mushrooms and Red Pepper*
Oven-Roasted Vegetables*
Berries with frozen, nondairy dessert topping
TOTAL CALORIES: 600

ROMANTIC MENU #2

The Kitchen Sink Vegetable Soup*
Pan-Fried Pork Chops with Fruit Chutney*
Lentils with a Twist*
Apple & Pear Parfait*
TOTAL CALORIES: 575

*See recipe section, pages 132–146

4. The Crowded House Years

WOMEN WHO ARE TRYING TO LOSE WEIGHT while caring for children often report that they can't find the time or energy to eat right or exercise. Many women say that they never lost those last 10 pounds after delivering their first child, and find themselves 20 pounds heavier after their second. Mothers who have adopted children may have bypassed the added pregnancy pounds, but still have to contend with the obstacles to weight loss that all moms confront.

The joys of motherhood are interspersed with many challenges. Interrupted sleep, 24/7 duty and not being able to find a free moment to think about your needs all make it difficult to remember whether or not you ate all your greens today. Heck, you have no idea *what* you ate today! You do, however, know in exacting detail what Junior ate, how much and when. Added to this new, larger-than-life workload for new moms is the emotional roller-coaster ride most find themselves on while molding their lives to include this new demanding role.

Moms with new babies and toddlers underfoot have the burden of attending to the daily, immediate needs of an impatient group of little people. Mothers with older kids struggle to keep up with packed after-school calendars. And those with both little ones and older children have the daunting task of juggling the older ones' social calendars while dragging along the younger kids.

No wonder women at this stage of life find that maintaining a healthy weight and engaging in an exercise program is close to impossible. I'll admit that there are a few women who seem to keep everything in order and exercise and eat right regardless of the chaos around them. Just knowing that these women exist can spark feelings of inadequacy and frustration in others trying to control their weight. Take comfort, though, in knowing that these women are the exception rather than the rule. I've spent countless hours counseling women who need some guidance and help in pulling together a healthier lifestyle. The question is, "Can I possibly turn things around in my life and find the time and energy to regain a healthier, leaner me?" Of course you can! Whether you're a new mother trying to lose those pregnancy pounds, a soccer mom racing from the kitchen to the game or a woman juggling the demands of corporate life with the needs of children, you can take charge and lose that excess weight. Use the suggestions, tips and guide sheets in this chapter to help you leap over your obstacles to living a healthier, leaner life.

BRAND-NEW MOM

You arrive home from the hospital with your bundle of joy in your arms. The world is a blessed and happy place. With a smile on your face, you place your baby in that beautiful new cradle. Then you contentedly proceed to your room and open the closet door. Your smile quickly fades as you realize, stricken, "There's nothing in there to wear!" You refuse to wear your maternity clothes (ugh!), but nothing else fits.

It's easy to get despondent when we place unrealistic expectations on ourselves. In one study, researchers at the University of Maryland followed 126 women right after childbirth for one year. They found that 70 percent of the women in the study were dissatisfied with their weight four months after delivery. At the baby's first birthday, 39 percent were still unhappy with their bodies. This dissatisfaction with body size was the cause of great frustration for many new moms, and was identified as one of the main factors that interfered with the resumption of sexual intimacy following childbirth.

I'm not suggesting that women should be satisfied with excess body weight caused by eating too many calories and inactivity. What I am suggesting is that any woman who has just had a baby be realistic in setting short-term weight-loss and lifestyle goals. Your body has just gone through an incredible journey. In your mind, the trip has ended and you want to get off this large-bodied plane. However, it'll take time for the jet to carefully taxi to

If you're breastfeeding your baby, you should not restrict calories. Many experts suggest that eating fewer than 1,800 calories a day can decrease the nutritional quality of your milk and may also reduce the quantity you produce. Once again, patience is of the utmost importance. Make the right food choices, eat with regularity and begin to exercise (with your doctor's approval). You can reduce calories to a lower level once you and your baby are ready for weaning.

the gate and unload all that baggage.

You can eat right, get more physical activity and lose weight in the months following childbirth. Just realize that your body needs your time, patience and understanding as it shrinks back to its pre-pregnancy size.

First of all, give yourself six weeks to adjust to your new baby and schedule. Your body needs extra rest and time to recuperate after delivery. There's no harm, and every benefit, in eating healthily during this time. I've prepared a snack list for new moms (page 65) to help you plan your day with healthy foods.

Stress and Weight Gain

Juggling many responsibilities at once is routine for most women, creating stress that's often present at all stages of a woman's life. However, "new mom" stress—along with the stress that comes with other happy, major life changes—ranks high on the stress scale. Most women are aware that stress will make you eat. There's a physical reason, as well as a psychological one, why stress pushes your hunger button. Hormonal changes set you up for increased physical hunger. Your stress hormone, cortisol (the one that gives you the "flight or fight" response during times of danger), rises in response to stress. This in turn triggers an insulin release from your pancreas. In Chapter 2 you learned that insulin will lay down fat and make you hungry. You don't want extra insulin in your body, but that's what happens when you're stressed. Stress cries out to be soothed. Food sometimes seems to be the only cure for what ails many new moms—especially late at night after a long, hard day with an infant. Of course, when you're trying to lose weight, indulging in a high-calorie treat leaves you feeling bad soon after the last bite. It's important that you begin to reward and comfort yourself with things that have nothing to do with food. "Treat" yourself to one of the following mom stress-busters next time you're having a day that sends you to the kitchen for a quick food fix.

Healthy Snacks for Busy New Moms

YOU'RE CRAVING	CHOOSE INSTEAD	COUNT AS	SAVE CALORIES
1 oz potato chips	3 cups microwave light popcorn	1 bread/starch	70
1 cup premium ice cream	1 cup lowfat frozen yogurt topped with 1 Tbsp chopped nuts*	1 bread/starch, 1 fat	270
5 chocolate chip cookies	3 graham cracker squares with 2 tsp peanut butter*	1 bread/starch, 1 fat	125
12 oz mocha-flavored coffee cooler	12 oz nonfat cappuccino**	1 dairy	150
Blueberry muffin	1 slice raisin toast with 1 Tbsp cream cheese	1 bread/starch, 1 fat	175
1½ oz chocolate bar	½ cup fat-free chocolate pudding	1 dairy	155
4 oz bagel with 2 Tbsp cream cheese	4 reduced-fat weave-type crackers with 1 oz reduced-fat cheese	1 bread/starch, 1 protein	250
10 tortilla chips with 2 Tbsp guacamole	2 celery sticks with 2 Tbsp hummus	1 vegetable, 1 fat	125

These snacks are also great choices when cravings are heightened during the days of PMS (premenstrual syndrome).

* If you're lactating and are concerned about possible future food allergies in your child, some doctors recommend not eating nuts or peanut butter.

** If you're lactating, decaffeinated cappuccino is recommended.

Stress-Busters for Moms

GO FOR A WALK. You'll be amazed how much better you feel after a breath of fresh air.

GIVE AN OLD FRIEND A CALL. Friends and family are your greatest resource when you're overwhelmed. Just chatting with someone who can lend a sympathetic ear will do wonders for your mood.

ACCEPT HELP WHEN OFFERED. It makes most people feel good when they can help a friend or family member. If people are offering to help, take them up on their offers. Be specific about what they can do. Have a friend fix you a healthy meal or watch the baby so you can take a quick nap and you'll feel better in no time at all.

TAKE A LONG SHOWER OR BATH. Light a candle and soak aching muscles.

READ A MAGAZINE OR A CHAPTER IN A NOVEL. Take a break from the baby-care books and feed your mind with things that spark different interests.

LISTEN TO RELAXING MUSIC. Put aside the lullabies and play the pre-baby music that you like once in a while.

WRITE YOUR FEELINGS DOWN IN A JOURNAL. Putting your thoughts down on paper allows you to put things in perspective. A journal will give you a place for release now, and you'll be able to preserve the memories of your baby's first days for a lifetime.

Keep Active

We all know how hard it is to find the time to exercise when you have a new baby in your home. Unfortunately, the physical rigors of taking care of a baby don't usually burn enough calories for weight loss. In addition, caring for your baby is demanding, and you need to exercise to relieve stress. With a little creativity you can squeeze in this essential activity. If you're having difficulty finding time to exercise, try some of the following strategies.

- Take the baby with you in the stroller for a walk. You'll both enjoy the change of scenery and fresh air, and you'll be burning calories.

- Ask your mate to take over for an hour so you can be free to exercise.

- Trade off babysitting with a trusted friend or neighbor, and use that time to exercise.

- Hire a mother's helper to watch your baby so you can exercise.

- Strength training can be done at home anytime. See Chapter 6 for details on exercise and equipment guidance.

- Join a mother's club that shares babysitting and provides programs that promote health and physical activity.

VETERAN MOM

YOU'VE BEEN PROVIDING COOKING, cleaning, recreational and tutoring services for children for some time now. You've come a long way since diaper-bag days, yet you still haven't been able to regain your slimmer, stronger body. Running the kids to and from activities, keeping the house in order, shopping for food, clothes and family gifts leave you drained by the end of the day. You literally drop into bed each night vowing to fit in a workout "tomorrow." You swear you'll plan and cook healthier meals "as soon as things get less hectic around here." Does all this sound far too familiar to you?

Don't beat yourself up because you haven't been able to accomplish your goals of exercising more and eating right. Anyone who has raised children knows what a demanding, important job it is. Often a mom needs to put her concerns and needs aside to provide for others. And yet it's time for a change—one that won't deprive the loved ones in your life, and one that will most definitely improve your physical and mental health. Remember that when you take good care of yourself, you'll be better equipped to take good care of others. It's also a great life lesson for your children to see you, their role model, eating right and exercising.

Let's start with exercise. You know how great you feel once you get moving. Let's carve some time out of your packed day and get those mood-enhancing endorphins flowing throughout your body. Keep in mind that any activity is better than none at all. You don't have to join an expensive gym or run a 5-K race to get the health and weight reduction benefits of increased physical activity.

Try These Creative Ways to Add More Physical Activity to Your Life

YOUR TYPICAL CALENDAR	WHAT YOU CAN DO INSTEAD
Junior has soccer practice.	Opt out of standing on the sidelines chatting with neighbors. Instead, take a long walk around the soccer field.
It's a rainy day, the kids are bored and so are you.	Pull out some jump ropes for you and the kids. Start jumping, going as slowly as you need to.
You're cleaning the house, always a drag.	Put on music that gets you moving, and dance around the tables as you dust them. Ignore the stares from your children.
It's Sunday afternoon and nothing much is going on.	Take the kids with you to the local high school track. You can walk on the track while the kids play catch in the center.
The kids are restless, and you're thinking of taking them to the movies.	Plan a more calorie-consuming activity. Take the kids to a skating rink, bowling alley or laser tag center. Make sure you join in the fun (and calorie-burning) activity, too.

MOM ON THE HOME FRONT

THE DAYS ARE LONG AND DEMANDING when you're home full time with children. The women I know who chose to be stay-at-home moms are happy with their decision and have no regrets. However, that doesn't mean their lives are free of the frustrations of being the full-time caregiver to youngsters. The hours are long, the job is messy and no one offers to cover for you at lunchtime. Often, stay-at-home moms feel that they don't get sufficient respect from husbands and others in their life for the important job they do. Let's face it, many people don't realize how demanding, time-consuming and difficult a job it is. Some people think since you're on the home front all day that you should take care of *everything*! (Of course, these are people who never held down your job.) Your life is as enriched as it is sometimes frustrating. You also confront obstacles to eating right and exercising that women with different jobs don't. Take a look at some of the most common obstacles that moms on the home front encounter, as well as some solutions to overcoming them.

Obstacles and Solutions to Eating Healthier for Moms on the Home Front

OBSTACLE	CAUSE(S)	SOLUTION(S)
You seem to have no time to prepare healthy, low-calorie meals.	The kids' schedules drain your day of any free time.	Plan a day to cook in bulk. Freeze extra for other nights. Have your mate or another adult watch the children.
	It's dangerous to cook with little ones underfoot.	Create a healthy meal swap with other moms and dads. Take turns cooking for both families (just double the recipes).
	The kids don't want to eat the healthy food you've cooked.	Get the kids involved in the meal preparation. They'll be more interested in eating the vegetables if they've rinsed them before you steam them. Have little ones set the table.
You always eat the leftover food on your kids' plates.	You were brought up to never waste food.	Remind yourself that you're eating leftover kiddie food: There's nothing appealing about that!
	You feel that since you're eating off their plates, not yours, the calories don't count.	Make sure you eat something healthy while your kids eat so you're not tempted by hunger to graze off their plates.
		If your child is old enough, have him or her scrape the leftover food into the garbage.
You find it particularly hard to resist treats in the evening. The kids are finally asleep and at last you can relax...and eat in peace.	Many people eat to relax. It seems a small, yet well-deserved, reward for a long, hard day.	Think of all the things you could do to reward yourself and unwind that have nothing to do with food.

OBSTACLE	CAUSE(S)	SOLUTION(S)
You can't find time during the day to sit down to a healthy meal, so you wind-up picking at food all day long.	Mealtimes at your house sometimes resemble a food fight. Who can eat a meal with all that going on?	Schedule time to take a break. Spend the time when the baby is napping, or when the kids are watching television, to sit down to a healthy meal.
Dinner seems to creep up on you. You never seem to find the time to plan meals in advance.	There just aren't enough hours in the day to do everything. The kids have you out of the house most of the day, leaving little time for meal preparation.	Make meal planning a priority. All it takes is an hour a week to plan your meals and make a grocery list. Having the right foods in the house and a weekly dinner schedule on the refrigerator make meal preparation easier.

MOM AT THE OFFICE

MAKING THE CHOICE, or having the choice made for you, to work outside the home while raising children is a mixed blessing. More and more women are juggling work and kids. In 1975, 45 percent of women with young children worked outside the home. By 1997 that number had shot up to 71 percent. The rewards of providing a service to people over 2 feet tall, who sometimes remember to say thank you, can be a great perk. However, you have responsibilities at home and demands from the people you report to at work. Is it the best of both worlds or an impossible schedule to face most days? Most working women find it difficult to just get through the day knowing that dinner preparation, laundry and bathtime await them at home. It makes it hard to find the energy to exercise and eat right. Use the solution chart on the next page to find some creative ways to tackle your obstacles to weight loss. Keep in mind that, just like moms on the home front, you need to find stress-reduction techniques that have nothing to do with food (see Stress-Busters for Moms, page 66). Make sure to schedule time just for you. This may take a lot of planning in the beginning, but soon taking better care of yourself will become routine.

Obstacles and Solutions to Eating Healthier for Moms at the Office

OBSTACLE	CAUSE(S)	SOLUTION(S)
You can't seem to get a healthy meal on the table in the evening after a long day at work.	There truly are not enough hours in the day sometimes.	Create healthy meals in a flash by combining ready-to-use foods with fresh foods. Buy a rotisserie chicken and microwave fresh steamed broccoli and sweet potatoes.
You have no time or energy in the evening to exercise.	Your days are long and you arrive home in the evening wanting to spend time with the kids. You also have to catch up on laundry and housecleaning.	Use your lunchtime to get in a bit of physical activity. Go for a half-hour walk after eating a quick lunch. Use your commuting time to exercise. Get off the bus one stop early and walk the rest of the way to your destination.
You feel overwhelmed by all you need to accomplish. This stops you from being active and productive.	Having too many responsibilities can immobilize you.	Invest an hour or so in planning a weekly schedule. Find a routine that works for you. Laundry on Mondays, exercise on Tuesdays, grocery shopping on Saturdays, and so on.
You find yourself eating high-fat lunches.	Everyone in the office is ordering pizza and Chinese food. You're really hungry and would love to eat it, too.	If you have a refrigerator at work, brown-bag your lunch. Make a turkey sandwich on whole-grain bread and toss in an apple. Or fill a plastic container with fresh salad and add a few ounces of leftover chicken breast and a teaspoon of lowfat dressing.

THE SINGLE MOM

If you're a single mom, no doubt you know that you're carrying a bigger burden than most mothers. Single-mom households are on the rise. In 1970, 10.7 percent of all new births were to single moms. That number increased to 32.4 percent in 1997. While divorce isn't on the rise, in 1997 one million divorces were granted. As a single mom, there isn't anyone else on the home front with whom to share the burden of child care. Whether it's an emotional or physical need that has to be attended to, you're the only one on deck, which takes an additional toll on you. Researchers have found that of all mothers interviewed, single moms have the poorest health. Recognize that you have a valid need for help, from friends, family and sitters, that will allow you to recharge your batteries.

It's obviously time to make a change for improved health. Let the people around you know that you're working on increasing your exercise time and trying to eat healthier. You'll probably find great support and encouragement from those in your life who care about you. Accept any help offered to make your plan for changing to a healthier life happen. Spend time working on incorporating nonfood stress-busters into your day.

FAST-FOOD DINING DILEMMAS SOLVED

As a busy mom, chances are you eat some meals at fast-food restaurants, like it or not. Either the kids are begging to go or you need to have dinner taken care of quickly. Having more meals out is one option that many moms take to get everything done before the sun goes down. Eating fast food doesn't have to be a diet disaster, though. Take a look at the fast-food guide to eating lower calorie and lower fat meals on page 73.

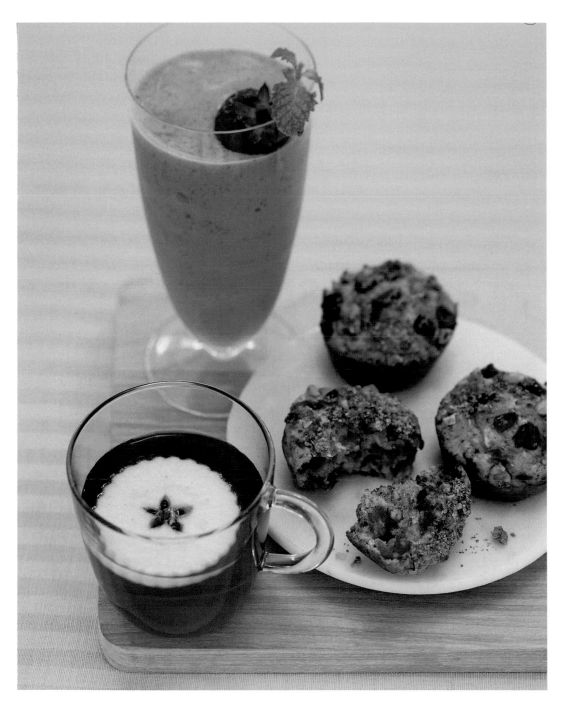

Breakfast Smoothie and Cranberry-Nut Muffins (page 132)
Hot Spiced Apple-Cranberry Cider (page 133)

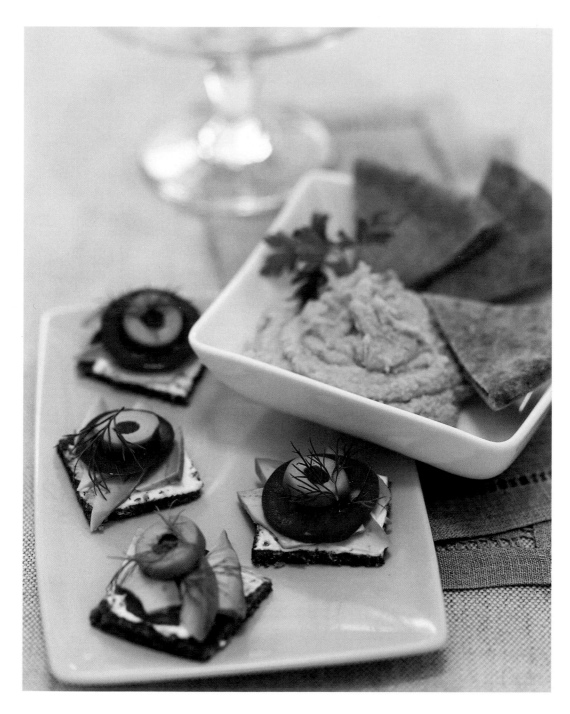

Herb and Avocado Canapés (page 133)
Quick Hummus and Pitas (page 134)

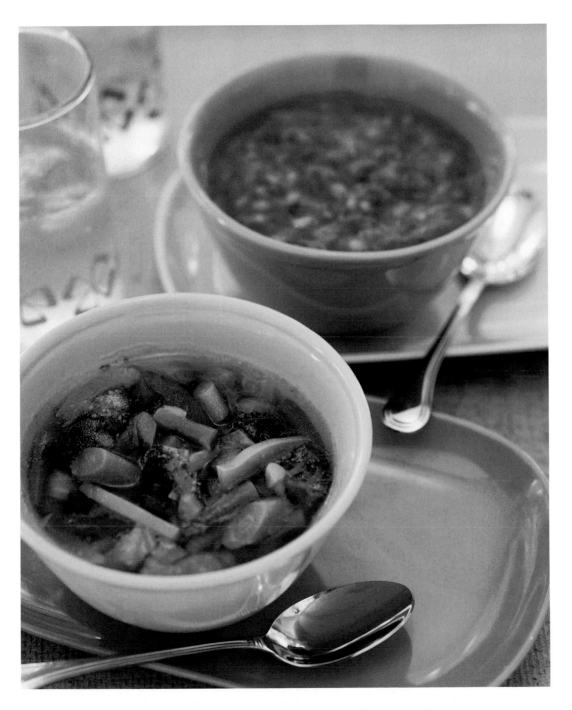

Tomato, Basil and Barley Bisque (page 134)
The Kitchen Sink Vegetable Soup (page 135)

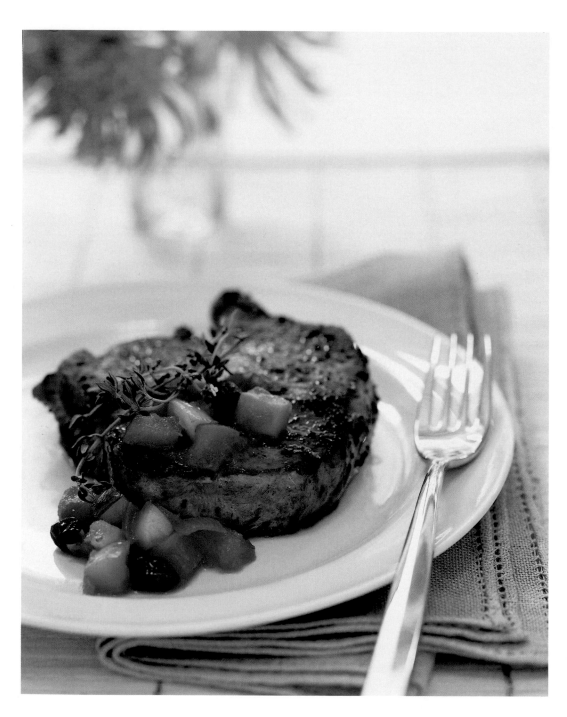

Pan-Fried Pork Chops with Fruit Chutney (page 135)

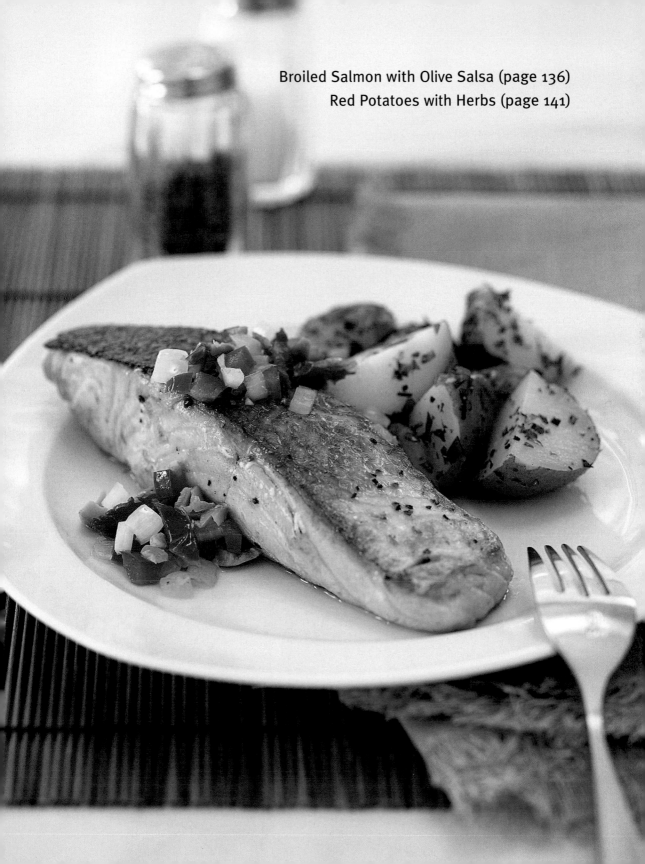

Broiled Salmon with Olive Salsa (page 136)
Red Potatoes with Herbs (page 141)

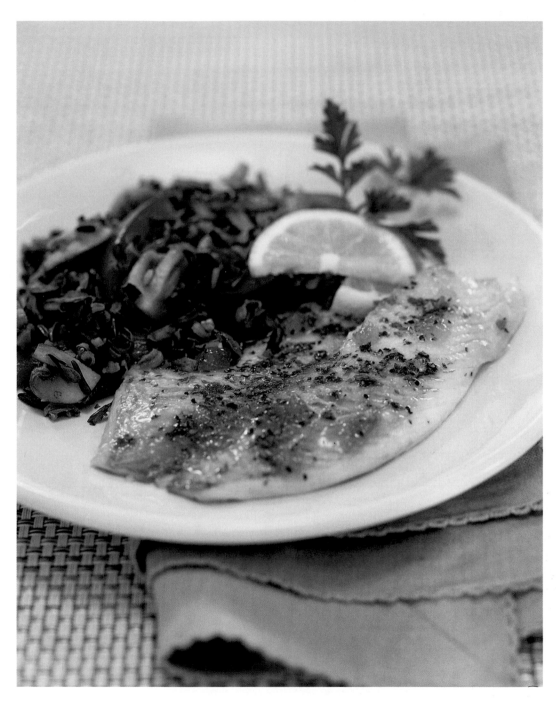

Apricot-Lemon Glazed Fish Fillets (page 136)
Wild Rice with Mushrooms and Red Pepper (page 140)

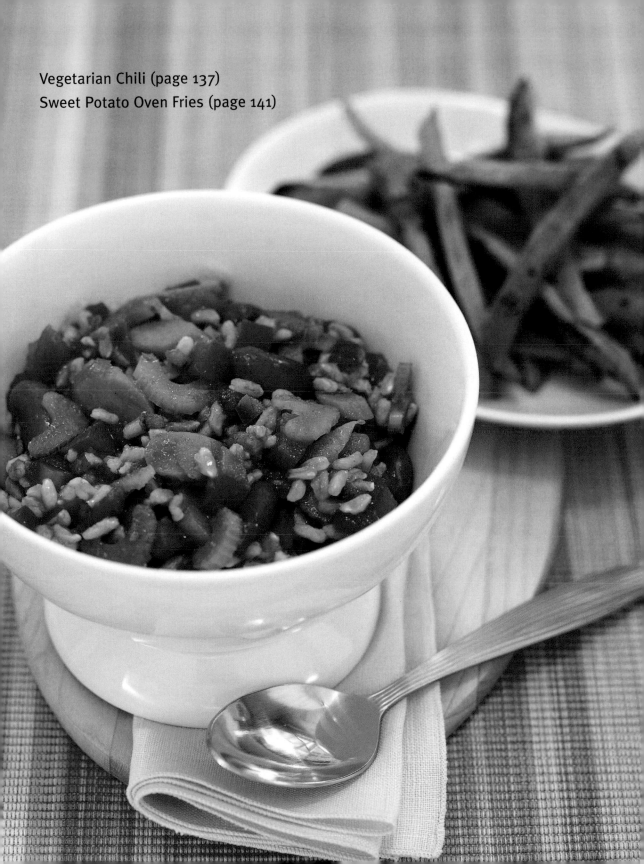

Vegetarian Chili (page 137)
Sweet Potato Oven Fries (page 141)

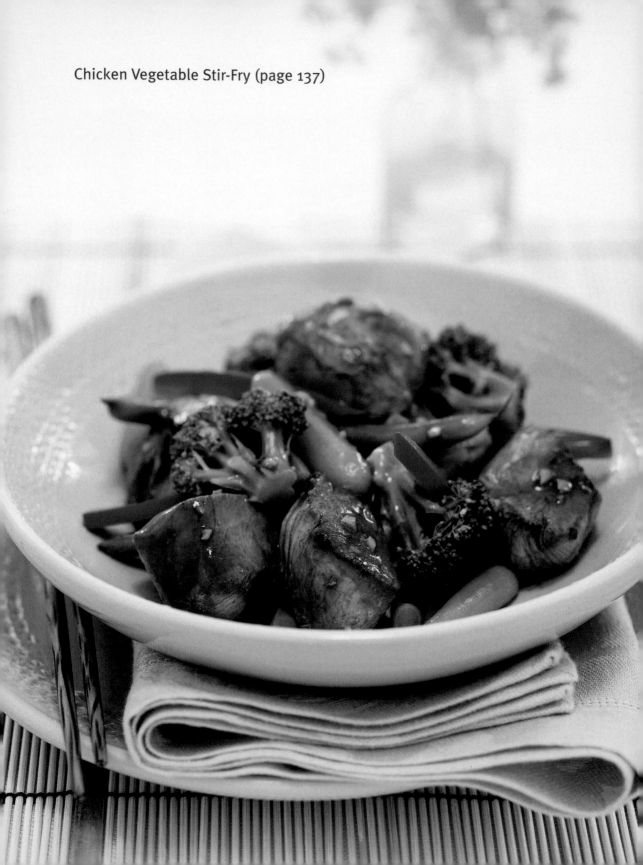

Chicken Vegetable Stir-Fry (page 137)

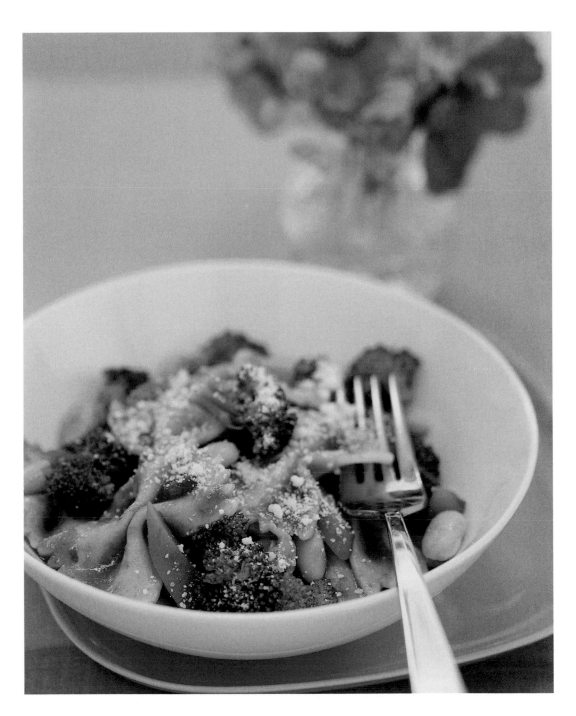

Bow-Tie Pasta with Beans and Vegetables (page 138)

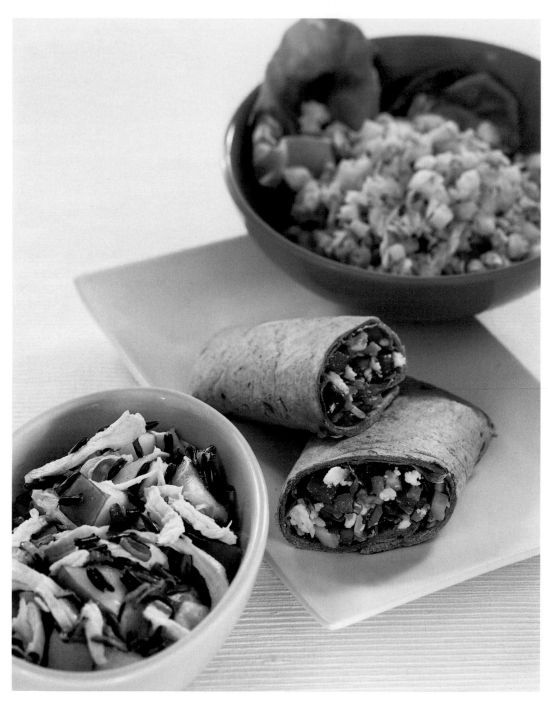

Tangy Tuna Salad and Feta Cheese Wrap (page 139)
Pear and Chicken Salad (page 138)

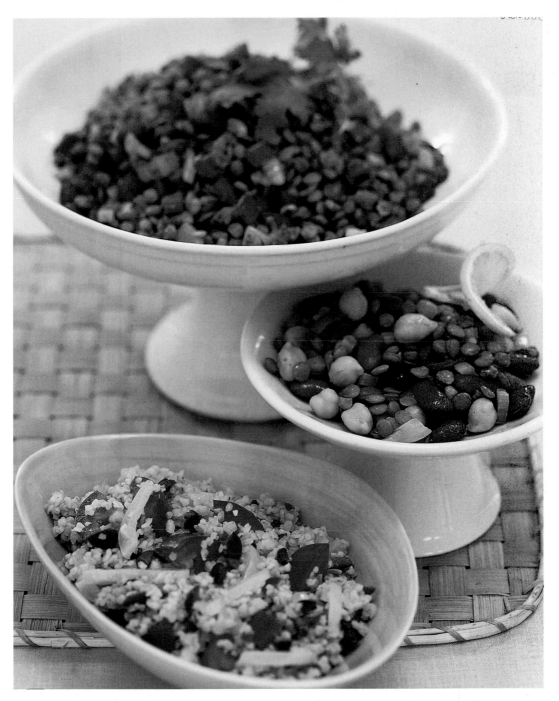

Lentils with a Twist (page 140) Cold Bean Salad (page 142)
Tasty Bulgur with Olives and Peppers (page 144)

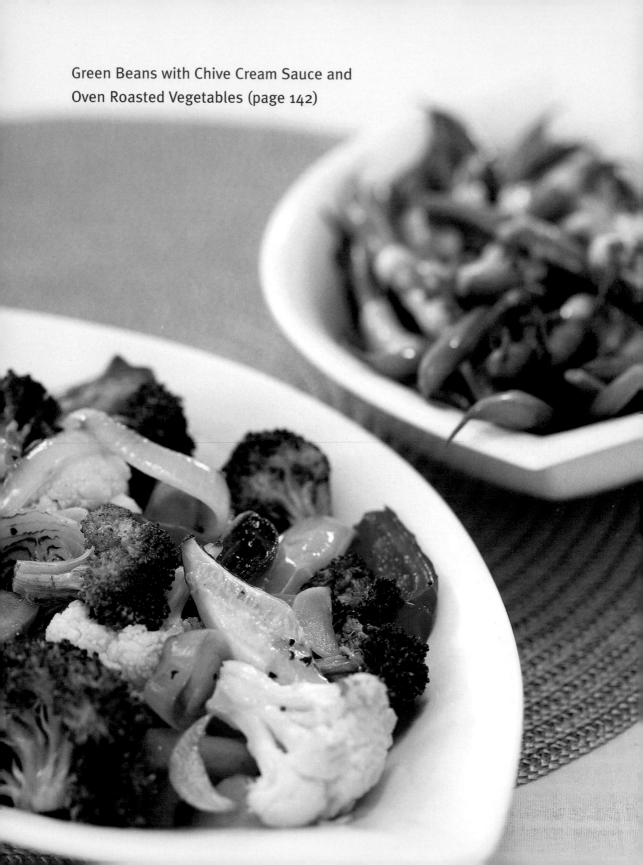

Green Beans with Chive Cream Sauce and
Oven Roasted Vegetables (page 142)

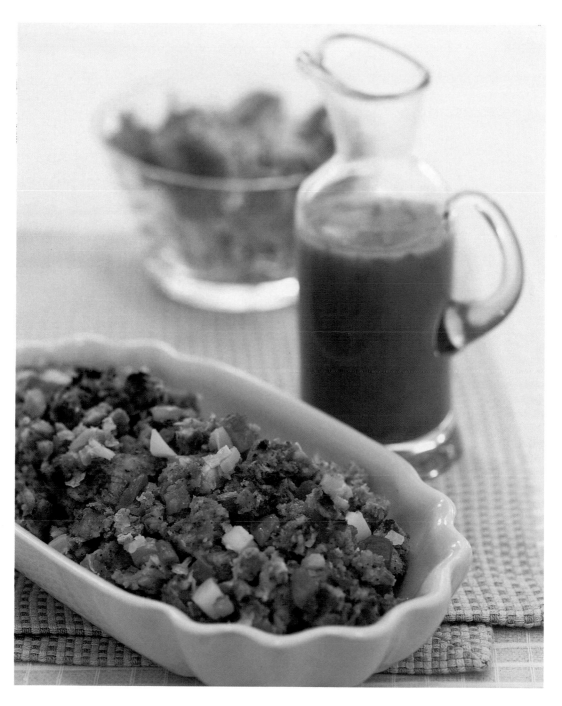

Tangy Vinaigrette Dressing and
Fruit Stuffing (page 143)

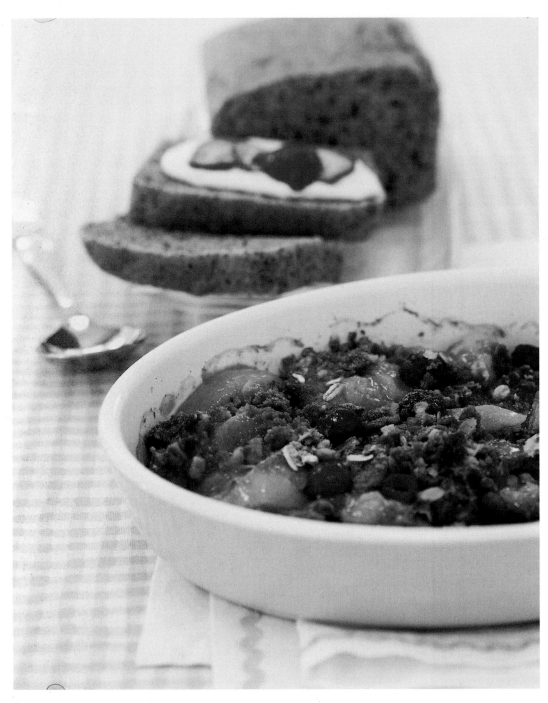

Flavorful Fruit Crisp (page 144)
Yogurt, Lemon and Poppy Seed Bread (page 145)

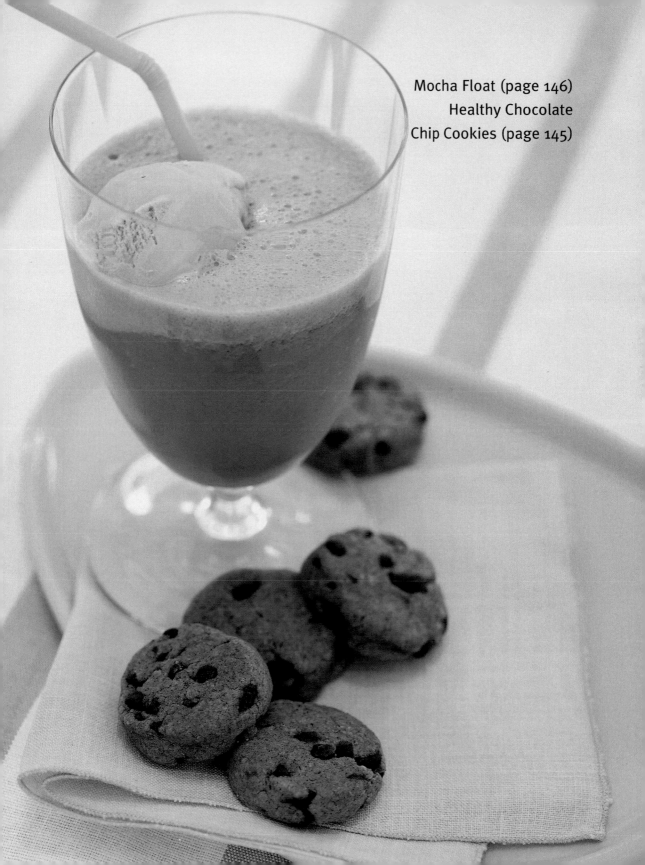

Mocha Float (page 146)
Healthy Chocolate
Chip Cookies (page 145)

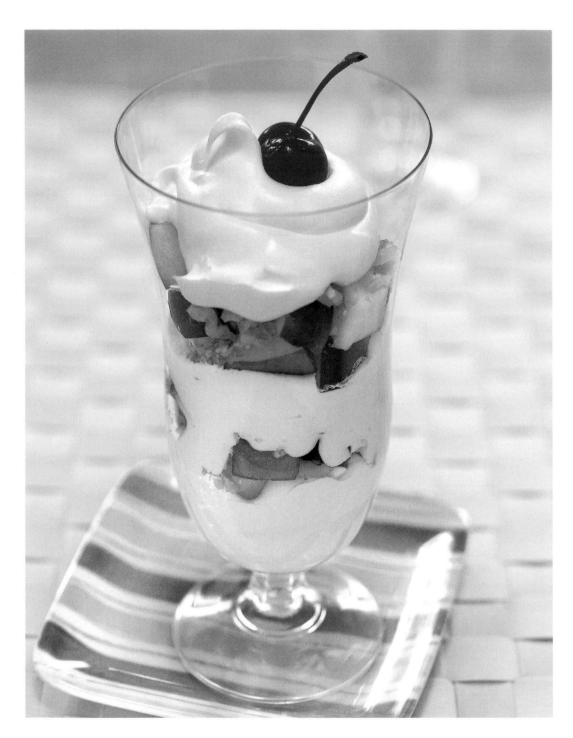

Apple and Pear Parfait (page 146)

Healthy Fast Food Choices

(LISTED IN ORDER OF INCREASING CALORIE CONTENT)

Many fast-food restaurants offer lower fat choices such as soups and vegetarian burgers. These food items are not yet provided nationally, so you need to check availability with restaurants in your area. Let managers know that there's a demand for these lower fat, lower calorie items.

BURGER KING		
CHOOSE	CALORIES/FAT	FOOD CHOICE SERVINGS
Broiled Chicken Salad with 1 oz reduced-calorie light Italian dressing	205/9 g	3 proteins, 1 fat, 2 vegetables
BK Broiler Chicken Sandwich (hold the mayonnaise) Side Salad with 1 oz reduced-calorie light Italian dressing	445/13 g	4 proteins, 2½ bread/starches, 1½ fat, 1 vegetable
Cheeseburger and side salad with 1 oz reduced-calorie light Italian dressing	455/23 g	3 proteins, 2 bread/starches, 3 fats, 1 vegetable
Small, plain hamburger, ½ serving small French fries	455/20 g	2 proteins, 3 bread/starches, 3 fats
PIZZA HUT		
CHOOSE	CALORIES/FAT	FOOD CHOICE SERVINGS
2 slices Veggie Lover's Pizza (Thin 'n' Crispy Crust)	340/12 g	2½ bread/starches, 2 fats, 2 vegetables
1 slice cheese pizza (hand-tossed) 1 plate greens and vegetables from the salad bar with 1 Tbsp fat-free dressing	355/13 g	2 proteins, 2 bread/starches, 2 fats, 1 vegetable
1 slice cheese pizza with ham (Sicilian-style), 1 plate greens and vegetables from the salad bar with 1 Tbsp fat-free dressing	365/13 g	2 proteins, 2 bread/starches, 2 fats, 1 vegetable
Spaghetti with marinara sauce (hold the garlic bread)	490/6 g	5 bread/starches, 1 fat, 2 vegetables

DENNY'S		
CHOOSE	CALORIES/FAT	FOOD CHOICE SERVINGS
(Breakfast Menu) Junior Waffle Supreme, 1 order Canadian bacon, 1½ oz reduced-calorie syrup, 1 serving fruit in season	360/16 g	2 proteins, 2 bread/starches, 2 fats, ½ fruit
8 oz split-pea soup, Grilled Alaskan Salmon Dinner (order with plain mashed potatoes and broccoli with butter)	515/13 g	4 proteins, 2½ bread/starches, 2 fats, 2 vegetables
Grilled Chicken Breast Dinner (order with baked potato and carrots in honey glaze), side Garden Salad (with 2 Tbsp fat-free honey-mustard dressing)	540/10 g	3 proteins, 3½ bread/starches, 1½ fats, 3 vegetables
Garden Chicken Delite Salad with 2 Tbsp reduced-fat French dressing ½ piece chocolate cake (share with a friend)	540/20 g	3 proteins, 3 bread/starches, 3 fats, 2 vegetables
TACO BELL		
CHOOSE	CALORIES/FAT	FOOD CHOICE SERVINGS
1 Soft Taco Supreme	260/14 g	1 protein, 1½ bread/starches, 2 fats
1 Gordita Fiesta Chicken	280/12 g	1 protein, 2 bread/starches, 2 fats
1 Tostado	300/15 g	1 protein, 2 bread/starches, 2 fats
1 Chilli Cheese Burrito	330/13 g	1 protein, 2½ bread/starches, 2 fats
2 Tacos	360/20 g	2 proteins, 2 bread/starches, 2½ fats

5. The Later Years

YOU'VE REACHED A STAGE OF LIFE when you finally know yourself well, and it feels good. You're happier, more relaxed and more focused than ever. You wouldn't trade your hard-earned wisdom and contentment for anything—except perhaps a younger, faster metabolism! It's a fact, not fiction, that your metabolism has also become more "relaxed" as the years have flown by. The reduction in your need for fuel is mainly due to your loss of muscle mass. This happens to men and women alike as we age. As you've read earlier in this book, muscle is more energy-needy than fat, so as you lose muscle, your body needs far fewer calories to maintain the same body weight.

In addition to a loss of muscle mass, you may be experiencing hormonal shifts that can wreak havoc on your weight (and your general sense of well-being). As if puberty (and perhaps childbirth) wasn't enough, now you have to contend with uncomfortable symptoms from a body that produces less estrogen and progesterone. You may also find yourself "sandwiched" between simultaneously meeting the needs of your children and your aging parents. Some reports show that 25 percent of all American households have at least one adult who has cared for an elder in the past year. Stress mounts as many caregivers have to pass up job promotions and lose contact with friends and other social support systems. It probably comes as no surprise that 73 percent of caregivers are women. The average age of caregivers is 46, with 50 percent working full time and 66 percent married, according to the National Alliance for Caregiving. When you're a caregiver, finding time to exercise and eat right may seem like an unobtainable goal.

As you age, joint pain, disability and a decline in energy can interfere with your ability to be as active as you've been in the past. You may be living alone now and have lost interest in cooking healthy meals for just yourself. The accumulated wisdom from life is wonderful, but you're getting really tired of carrying around those extra pounds.

Women in the later stages of life, even those in the throes of menopause, can successfully lose weight. What does it take to lose weight at this stage? You simply need to become more physically active and find ways to creatively cut calories. Patience is also essential, because you can't lose weight at the same rate you did in your 20s. But lose you will!

THROUGH PERIMENOPAUSE AND BEYOND

YOU'RE CONSIDERED MENOPAUSAL when you haven't had a period for more than a year and there's no other reason for the cessation of your menses. The perimenopausal stage is the period of time between when menstrual cycles change and become irregular until menopause. This stage can last for several years, and it can be a frustrating and difficult time. Hormonal levels during the perimenopausal phase may not reveal a reduction in hormonal secretion, yet you may in fact be experiencing distressing symptoms of perimenopause.

The average age for perimenopause is 47½, and the average age for menopause is 51. The symptoms of natural menopause develop slowly and intensify with time. However, women with surgically induced menopause (when both ovaries are removed) or chemically induced menopause (from chemotherapy) experience a dramatic drop in estrogen, triggering a severe onset of menopausal symptoms.

SYMPTOMS OF PERIMENOPAUSE INCLUDE

- Irregular periods
- Hot flashes
- Bloating/weight gain
- Dizziness/loss of coordination
- Irritability
- Depression
- Night sweats/sleep disturbance
- Vaginal dryness/decrease in libido

We really don't know as much as we should about the perimenopausal years. Studies are underway to find better ways to intervene and help woman in perimenopause. In one study conducted at the

University of Pennsylvania Medical Center, researchers investigated reports of symptoms of perimenopause in women between ages 35 and 47. They interviewed 436 healthy women who were not taking antidepressants or oral contraceptives and were not on hormone replacement therapy, who had menstrual cycles in the normal range (every 22 to 35 days) for three months prior to the start of the study, and who had an intact uterus and ovaries.

Researchers found that 37 percent of the women reported menopausal symptoms. Thirty percent reported experiencing hot flashes, the symptom typically viewed as the true sign of menopause. The data is significant because the average age of the study participant was 41, a full decade earlier than the average age for the onset of menopause. African-American women in the study reported an even higher percentage of symptoms (46 percent).

Clearly, perimenopausal symptoms play a hand in how women feel well before menopause begins. But multiple research studies have debunked the belief that menopause or hormone replacement therapy is the cause for weight gain at this stage of life. However, researchers have found that there is a redistribution of fat to the waist area in perimenopausal and menopausal women, which increases a woman's waistline by about an inch.

I've counseled enough women in their 40s and 50s to know that they don't care what the research reports: They know that they're having difficulty losing weight or maintaining a healthy weight, and they're certain that the hormonal changes they're experiencing are somehow to blame. With sleep disturbances, hot flashes, irritability and vaginal dryness, who wouldn't be cranky and stressed? And we know that stress causes weight gain. The stress hormone, cortisol, increases in response to stress, which in turn increases insulin—that nasty hormone that makes you hungry and helps you lay down fat. So menopause may indirectly cause weight gain because of its accompanying stress, but not because of hormonal shifts. Sleep deprivation, irritability, bloating and mild depression may also lead to inactivity and overeating.

What Can I Do to Lose Weight When My Body Wants to Do the Opposite?

THE BEST WAY TO LOSE WEIGHT despite your changing hormones, decreasing muscle mass and higher stress and cortisol levels is to exercise. Working on ways to reduce stress and finding time for rest will also go a long way in helping you reduce your food intake. Sleep deprivation and stress are strong hunger triggers. If you're sleep-deprived because of night sweats, try to grab a 15- to 20-minute nap during the day. Reduce stress by taking a break from the office or your usual routine and go for a walk, read a book or listen to your favorite music on a portable player.

Exercising consistently ranks as an important factor in losing weight and in maintaining weight loss. Research finds that exercise is also an especially powerful component in reducing the symptoms women feel during perimenopause. In one study conducted at Loyola University in Chicago, researchers reported that in a group of 214 women aged 40 to 55, exercise reduced menopausal symptoms significantly. Women who were relatively active reported far fewer incidences of irritability, forgetfulness, headache, vaginal dryness and decreased libido than women who were less active. Here are some ways to pump up your exercise program during menopause.

Ways to Increase Your Exercise Time

FIND AN EXERCISE BUDDY. Walk—and talk—with a friend. Most women feel better after venting frustrations. Why not take the time to exercise while unloading your problems?

MARK YOUR CALENDAR. Many people plan on exercising "this week," but before they know it, the week is over. By simply scheduling the time to exercise, the likelihood of it happening increases dramatically.

KEEP A LIST OF THE BENEFITS OF EXERCISE HANDY. Weight loss, improved sleep and reduction of heart-disease risk and menopausal symptoms are all benefits of exercise. Post the list prominently in your home or office as a frequent reminder.

FIND A HOBBY THAT INVOLVES PHYSICAL ACTIVITY. Hopefully, menopause is a phase of life when you'll be able to find the time to explore new and interesting hobbies. If you are physically up to it (and your doctor approves, of course) try learning a new sport such as golf, swimming, tennis or cross-country skiing.

MENOPAUSE AND INCREASED RISK OF ILLNESS

WOMEN ARE AT GREATER RISK of developing heart disease, osteoporosis and breast cancer once menopause starts. The protective benefits of estrogen—which help maintain a heartier bone mass density and lower cholesterol levels—are no longer present. We know that total and LDL (bad) cholesterol levels rise as estrogen levels fall, but few studies have given us data on just how much of a rise we can expect. One small long-term study gives us some insight into what happens to the levels of fat in our blood during menopause.

In a seven year study conducted in Japan, 16 healthy women aged 47 to 56, who steered clear of hormonal or herbal intervention, were followed for four years prior to, and three years following, menopause. Researchers observed the changes in blood levels of fat that are associated with increased risk of heart disease. Results revealed that during the study period, total cholesterol rose by 25 mg (14 percent) and LDL (bad) cholesterol increased by 20 mg (19 percent). Triglycerides and HDL (good) cholesterol remained virtually unchanged. Researchers concluded that these changes in fat levels were significant enough to increase the risk of plaque formation in perimenopausal women.

During menopause, bone density begins to decline. In one study of 290 premenopausal women done at the University of Pittsburgh, researchers noted declining bone mineral density at the onset of perimenopausal symptoms. While women aged 44 to 50 who had irregular menstrual cycles had a greater rate of bone loss at the spine and hip than women who reported no symptoms of menopause, this latter group of women still had significant bone loss. This evidence points to the need to include more calcium-rich foods in your diet, or to use calcium supplements before menopause sets in (see Chapter 3, page 51 for a list of calcium-rich foods).

In an interesting study reported in the *American Journal of Medicine* (April 2002), researchers at the University of Auckland in New Zealand found that calcium supplementation in postmenopausal women (average age 72) not only aids bone health but may improve cholesterol levels, too. In the study of 223 women, half were given 1,000 mg of calcium citrate daily while the other half received a placebo. At the end of one year, the calcium-treated group had a 7 percent increase in their HDL (good) cholesterol levels and a 6 percent reduction in the LDL (bad) cholesterol readings.

The risk of developing breast cancer increases as we age, so this is another big concern for women during the menopause years. Hormone replacement therapy (HRT) may increase the risk of developing hormone-dependent cancers (breast and endometrial), so women with a personal or family history of breast cancer are not usually candidates for HRT. Research shows that a better diet and increased exercise can aid in reducing breast cancer risk. Increasing exercise, eating more omega-3 fatty acid–rich foods (such as fatty fish, flaxseeds and walnuts) and more whole grains and fiber-rich foods, as well as reducing the intake of saturated fats, are all associated with reducing breast cancer risk. In a report published in the *Journal of the American College of Nutrition*, researchers at the University of Minnesota looked at the impact whole-grain foods has on decreasing cancer risk. They found that whole grains are rich in antioxidants, trace minerals, fiber and phytoestrogens (in the form of lignin), and they also slow down glucose response, which decreases circulating insulin levels. Recent studies suggest that high insulin levels may actually increase certain body chemicals that promote tumor growth, particularly in endometrial, colorectal and breast cancer. So eating whole grains is wise for women who want to reduce their risk of developing cancer. An added bonus: The extra fiber helps you lose weight, too. Consider replacing your typical grains with the healthier, higher fiber choices (see *below*).

Eat More Healthy Whole Grains		
INSTEAD OF	CHOOSE	INCREASE DIETARY FIBER BY (GRAMS)
2 slices white bread	2 slices branola-type bread	4
1 cup white rice	1 cup bulgur wheat	7
Large white-flour roll	1 whole-wheat pita pocket	2
1 cup cornflakes	1 cup 100% bran-flake cereal	5
TOTALS		18

What About HRT?

FOR YEARS MANY WOMEN HAVE BEEN DUTIFULLY TAKING HRT, believing they were doing more good than harm. So the results from the Women's Health Initiative study released in April 2002 sent shock waves through the medical and patient communities. Researchers were investigating the health benefits versus the risks of the most commonly used combined hormone preparation in the U.S., estrogen plus progestin, and planned to follow more than 16,000 women aged 50 to 79 for eight and a half years. However, the study was halted a little after five years when it was found that women who took estrogen plus progestin had a higher incidence of blood clots, coronary heart disease and breast cancer than those who took a placebo pill.

The news sent many women scrambling to find alternatives. Unfortunately, there are no quick and easy answers on the subject. In fact, there seem to be more questions than answers about herbal remedies as replacements for HRT for perimenopausal and menopausal women. In the meantime, there is some information to help you make informed choices.

Keep in mind that just because something is "natural" doesn't mean it can't harm you. Herbs, or any natural substances, taken in excess can be potentially harmful. Be as cautious with herbal remedies as you would any drug you'd ingest daily. Talk to your doctor or to a dietitian before taking any herbal remedy to be sure you're well informed about all the potential risks and benefits. Tell your doctor about any herbs you're already taking, as some may interfere with prescription medication.

Before we talk about specific herbs you need to know a bit about the mechanism of action of these herbs. The following terms will help explain the ways the various herbs work.

FREE RADICALS are the by-product created by the body's cells as they process oxygen. Free radicals damage cells and are implicated in the initiation and progression of disease. Environmental pollutants, chemicals and nitrates in food increase our exposure to free radicals.

ANTIOXIDANTS are protective substances that derail the potential damage caused by free radicals and are believed to help prevent cancer and heart disease. Vitamin A, vitamin C, vitamin E, beta-carotene and selenium are examples of nutrients that have antioxidant properties.

PHYTOCHEMICALS are chemicals found in many plant foods that aid in countering the effects of free radicals. There are thousands of phytochemicals in plants that are thought to aid in avoiding illnesses. Onions, garlic, citrus fruits, flaxseeds, berries, whole grains and broccoli are examples of phytochemical-rich foods.

PHYTOESTROGENS are a type of phytochemical. They are plant-based hormones that display estrogenlike activity because their structural components are similar to human estrogen. Phytoestrogens can be found in soybeans, grains, fruits and nuts.

Below are a few commonly recommended herbs and natural products with potential for use by menopausal women.

SOY

Soy products have received the greatest amount of attention and investigation as a natural source to aid in reducing menopausal symptoms, as well as the risk of cardiovascular disease, osteoporosis and breast cancer.

Much of the early research on soy products was based on epidemiological or observational data. Lower rates of reported menopausal symptoms, cardiovascular disease and breast cancer were observed in populations who consumed a diet rich in soy products. However, it may be that women who eat more soy products also tend to exercise regularly, don't smoke and eat more than the average amounts of fiber-rich foods. The question becomes, which of these variables—soy intake, increased exercise, not smoking, or eating a fiber-rich diet—is responsible for the reduction in menopausal symptoms, lower breast cancer and cardiac incidence? That's why the medical community prefers to use data from controlled clinical trials before making general recommendations to the public. In controlled trials, researchers compare the substance under study to a group taking a placebo (sugar pill). Researchers also hand select the participants they'll follow during the study and can therefore control individual variables that can skew the final results. These studies are expensive and take lots of time before results are made available to the public, but most agree controlled trials are worth the extra money and time involved. Results from controlled clinical trials provide us better direction, but not necessarily absolutes, in health care options. Many studies may report conflicting results that muddy the waters. Multiple trials confirming prior study results are your best guide when making decisions about changing lifestyle habits or food choices.

Controlled clinical trials investigating the health benefits of supplementation with phytoestrogens, often using soy products, have yielded different results. When soy was researched under controlled conditions, many researchers found little, if any, benefit in the soy-treated group versus the placebo group. There are conflicting reports about soy's role in lowering cholesterol levels. The studies that find a reduction in cholesterol with soy consumption report that the effect is minimal. The story is the same for soy's ability to reduce menopausal symptoms and prevent osteoporosis. Some see a small reduction of symptoms, while other studies don't find any benefit over the placebo-treated group. Many researchers believe that soy needs to be consumed for many years, perhaps beginning in adolescence, before it will provide the alleged health benefits.

Of more concern than the conflicting study results on soy's benefits is its potential to cause harm in high doses. Some investigators found an increased incidence in breast cancer in women treated with high doses of soy extracts. It seems the key here is quantity. The phytoestrogens in soy may aid in reducing breast cancer risk when taken in small amounts. However, phytoestrogens taken in large quantities—usually when consumed as an extract or powder—may actually increase the risk of breast cancer development by providing too much circulating estrogen.

In addition to concern about high soy intake and an increased breast cancer risk, other data have emerged questioning whether soy could be harmful in other ways. Recently, an association was noted between regular tofu consumption and an increased incidence of memory loss in women. Researchers found that women who ate tofu twice a week scored lower on memory tests than women who didn't eat it regularly. Researchers wonder if soy could somehow increase the rate at which the brain ages.

Until the evidence supporting the safety and usefulness of soy is more absolute, doctors recommend caution in adding soy to your diet. If you decide to include soy in your diet, it's best to consume it in its natural form— soy milk, tempeh, tofu or soybeans. Many health care experts recommend avoiding soy extracts, isoflavone supplements and isolated daidzein and genestein until the jury of researchers reaches a final verdict.

BLACK COHOSH

Black cohosh (*Cimicifuga racemosa*) is a large woodland plant native to eastern North America. Black cohosh was used by Native Americans and early settlers for snakebite, malaria and rashes. More than 100 years ago it was packaged as a treatment for "women's complaints." Today, black cohosh is touted as an aid in easing menopausal discomforts. German research supports the usefulness of black cohosh in reducing hot flashes and sleep disturbance. In one study of 629 women, researchers reported that 80 percent of women who took 40 mg a day of the black cohosh product Remifemin had a significant reduction in menopausal symptoms such as hot flashes within four weeks of taking the herb. Another German study found that taking more than 40 mg a day was no more effective than the standard dose in relieving menopausal symptoms. Additionally, they found that black cohosh appears to work without affecting estrogen, which implies that it does not increase the risk of hormone-dependent cancers (breast and endometrial). However, some investigators believe that the German studies were too small, uncontrolled and brief and could not reliably predict possible long-term adverse side effects of taking black cohosh.

A study conducted in the U.S. and reported in the March/April 2002 issue of *Menopause* looked at the potential for some herbs to stimulate human breast cancer cell growth. Researchers reported that black cohosh did not cause an increase in the growth of breast cancer cells under investigation as compared to untreated control cells, which would support the claim that it does not increase estrogenlike compounds in the body. In another trial conducted at Columbia University and the Weill-Cornell Medical College in New York City, 69 breast cancer survivors were given either a placebo or black cohosh to reduce hot flashes. The women in the study were asked to keep a four-day hot flash diary at the start of the study and at the one- and two-month marks. Researchers found no significant difference in hot flash reports between the group given black cohosh and the placebo-treated group. Interestingly, in retrospect both groups reported a perceived reduction in the number of hot flashes at the end of the study when compared to the beginning. Talk about a placebo effect!

When results are mixed, as they are here, it's best to discuss with your doctor the pros and cons of herbal treatment for menopausal symptoms. Side effects from black cohosh are typically mild gastric complaints. However, high doses can cause headache, vomiting and dizziness. If you decide to take black cohosh, keep in mind that the herb hasn't been studied for longer than six months at a time, so some health care professionals recommend taking it for no longer than that.

VITAMIN E

Taking high-dose vitamin E has been suggested as another natural alternative for diminishing uncomfortable menopausal symptoms. Again, the results of clinical trials are discouraging. In a study conducted at the Mayo Clinic in Minnesota, more than 100 breast cancer survivors were given 800 mg of vitamin E for four weeks and a placebo for four weeks. Participants kept daily hot flash diaries during the trial. Diaries did show that when the women were given vitamin E, they experienced one less hot flash a day than when they were given a placebo. However, researchers deemed this reduction in hot flash frequency marginally beneficial.

The Final Analysis

It's apparent that there are no clear answers to questions about treating menopausal symptoms or decreasing the risk of illness with natural remedies. However, most researchers believe that the use of phytoestrogens and other herbal remedies holds promise in improving health and in helping women through perimenopause and beyond. Research on phytoestrogens and other herbs is in its infancy and requires many more studies before we can say with certainty that these substances are safe and effective. Remember, the man behind the counter at the local health food store is not your best source for advice on natural remedies for menopause. Discuss all your options with a qualified health care professional.

Remedies That Work

I've devised a chart of the dietary and lifestyle habits that are strongly recommended in the scientific literature to alleviate perimenopausal symptoms and
avert illness.

HEALTH CONCERN	WHAT WORKS	WHAT TO DO
Menopausal discomfort	• Exercise	• Get moving and maintain a structured weekly exercise plan.
Osteoporosis	• Exercise • Calcium	• Do both aerobic and strength-training exercises. • Drink milk or calcium-fortified soy milk. Eat cheese or calcium-fortified soy cheese. Add calcium supplements to diet if needed (refer to Chapter 3 for daily calcium needs and a calcium counter).
Heart Disease	• Exercise • Weight loss • Lower intake of saturated fats • Omega-3 fatty acids • Vitamin E • Fiber-rich foods • Calcium	• Plan a weekly exercise agenda. • Make realistic weight goals and start cutting calories. • Limit high-fat cuts of meat. Eat more fish, chicken and turkey. • Eat fish, particularly salmon or sardines. Use canola oil or flaxseed oil and add flaxseeds to foods when possible.* • Talk to your doctor about supplementing your diet with vitamin E. • Choose high-fiber cereals, grains, fruits and vegetables. • Drink milk, eat reduced-fat cheese or take calcium supplements.

HEALTH CONCERN	WHAT WORKS	WHAT TO DO
Breast Cancer	• Exercise • Lower intake of fatty foods • Lower intake or elimination of alcohol • Omega-3 fatty acids	• Find exercise that you enjoy so you're motivated to be active most days of the week. • Choose lean meats; avoid saturated and trans-fatty acids. • Alcohol increases estrogen levels, which increase breast cancer risk. If you drink, do so in moderation (no more than 1 drink a night). • Eat fish, particularly salmon or sardines; use canola oil in salad dressing. Use 1 Tbsp flaxseed oil or add 1 Tbsp ground flaxseed to food daily.*

*If you are a breast cancer survivor you should talk to your doctor before consuming any phytoestrogen-rich food.

THE SENIOR YEARS

MAYBE YOU'VE JUST RETIRED or slowed down a bit on the job. Maybe you now have more leisure time and more time for your friends and family. These wonderful changes are the reason why some refer to the senior years as golden years. However, this less-hectic, less-structured time of life can contribute to weight gain. Many of my senior patients tell me they now eat out of boredom or because they have 24-hour access to the refrigerator!

Chances are that over the years you've experienced an injury or two, or maybe arthritis has taken its toll on you, and you've become less active. Add all this to a declining metabolism and you've got the explanation for why you may be having trouble losing those extra pounds at this stage of life. All you really need to do to successfully lose weight is make some adjustments in your lifestyle. Think of it as fine-tuning a picture to bring it into focus—and what a fine picture it will be once the adjustments are complete.

Exercise Is Key

Exercise is the main ingredient in the old-fashioned recipe for health and emotional contentment throughout your life. Research indicates that this is especially true in the later years. A 2001 report outlined in *Women's Health Issues* stated that in women over 60 there was a strong positive association between increased physical activity levels and an improved quality of life. The *Journal of the American Medical Association* reported that higher body weight can increase disability rates in middle-aged and older women. Women with a body mass index over 27 had a twofold increase in the risk of disability compared with women in the low body mass index group. At this stage of life lack of exercise and weight gain can become a vicious cycle. Added weight decreases your mobility, which causes you to gain more weight, which causes you to be even less active. Let's turn things around—slowly and with your physician's approval—and sneak some physical activity into your day. Most women who haven't exercised in years are surprised to find that small increases in physical activity can really improve their health and mood.

Exercise Tips for Seniors

I'm sure you have aches and pains in places you never knew existed. At least that's what many of my senior patients tell me. They also tell me that once they get started moving more, they feel so much better—healthier, more energetic and more powerful. I guess the research data hold true in the real world.

Sometimes it takes creativity to find ways to move more during the senior years. I've listed some ways to increase activity that have worked for many of my patients. However, you may have special considerations at this stage of life, and you should speak with your physician or a physical therapist for more individualized guidance.

WAYS FOR SENIORS TO SNEAK IN SOME EXERCISE

WALK WHENEVER YOU CAN. During inclement weather, walk around the shopping mall.

DO SOME STRENGTH TRAINING WHILE SITTING DOWN. Many seniors can build muscle mass by doing leg extensions and arm lifts while sitting down. The weight of your legs or arms creates enough resistance to increase muscle mass with movement. If you can, use light one-pound weights that you can strap around your ankles or wrists to increase the resistance.

USE 1-PINT WATER BOTTLES OR CANS AS FREE WEIGHTS to do strength training exercises if you don't belong to a gym or don't have any exercise equipment at home.

WATER AEROBICS is a great way for many seniors to exercise without stressing painful joints.

Vacation Plans Anyone?

If you're like many of the senior patients I see in my office, you like to travel. These later years often allow for more time to see the world. If you don't plan in advance, vacations can drill Swiss cheese–like holes in your plans for a healthier diet. Use the chart on the next two pages to stay on course, whether you're traveling the globe or just visiting the next town over.

Vacation Diet Dilemmas Solved		
VACATION DIET DILEMMA	**POTENTIAL PROBLEM**	**CORRECTIVE ACTION**
The extended time spent at the airport leaves you few healthy food options.	• Airport food is typically high in fat and calories. • Airlines no longer serve food on flights of less than three hours, so you have to eat something before you board.	• Eat a light meal before you leave for the airport. • Pack cottage cheese and fruit or a turkey sandwich to eat at the airport. • Look for chicken and salad at the airport. Use very little of the packaged dressing provided. • Look for a food stand that serves hearty soup. Choose bean or lentil soup and add two breadsticks. • Pack a protein bar.

VACATION DIET DILEMMA	POTENTIAL PROBLEM	CORRECTIVE ACTION
You eat only twice a day: a big breakfast and a huge dinner.	• You get too hungry before dinner and lose control at the meal. You slow your metabolism down by eating too infrequently.	• Be sure to take the time to eat lunch—even a light meal will do, such as yogurt and fruit or soup and a salad.
You allow seven to eight hours between your light lunch and dinnertime.	• If you let more than five hours lapse between meals, you'll be ready to eat the tablecloth at dinnertime.	• Carry snack food with you so you can have something healthy on the run. Protein bars, fruit and nuts or an ounce of cheese and some high-fiber crackers are good choices.
Driving to your destination takes time and you need to stop on the road for a meal.	• High-fat fast food and sweet treats are all around you.	• Pack a small cooler with healthy sandwiches and diet drinks. • Take a break at a scenic rest stop to eat your healthy meal.
Vacation time has always been a time for you to lie back, relax and indulge in food and drink.	• Overdoing it with food and drink will not only add too many calories to your diet, but make you feel out of control, leading to more overeating.	• Plan on one small indulgence every day while on vacation and stay on track the rest of the day. For example, one day you may choose to have a dessert after dinner, and the next day you may choose to have a higher calorie dinner entrée as your indulgence. All other choices during the day should be low calorie and healthy.
There's no exercise room in your hotel room.	• You want to stay on track with your exercise plan, but don't know the area you're in and aren't comfortable walking around town.	• Pack exercise bands to do some strength training in your hotel room. • Ask if there are any walking tours in the city you're visiting. • Before you leave, check with the hotel to see if there's a VCR in your room. If so, take an exercise tape with you.

Cooking for One

Many of my senior patients tell me that they spent much of their younger years cooking for a large family. It often included their husband and children, and sometimes their own mother or father, too. They find it impossible to cook for "just one person." However, that "just one person" is you, and you're important enough to plan and prepare a healthy meal for. Heck, you cooked all those years for everyone else—who deserves a healthy meal more than you do? Dining out and buying takeout food too frequently is a surefire way to overdo it with fat and calories. Use the cooking-for-one tips below to plan the meals your body deserves.

MAKE A SPECIAL MEAL FOR A SPECIAL PERSON: YOU

- Many meat items come prepackaged with two to four servings. Just buy the smallest size available and freeze the extra portion(s).

- Recipes that serve four can be cut in half without any detriment to the final product. Refrigerate half for later in the week, or freeze and date half the meal for a future date.

- Prepare a beautiful place setting for your meal. Put a tablecloth on the table, use your favorite china and light candles.

- Make mealtime special. Play relaxing music and let the answering machine pick up your calls.

PART THREE

Pulling It All Together

6. Exercise the Weight Off

YOU'VE GOT TO MOVE TO LOSE. It's that simple. Exercise is one of the most valuable weapons in your fight to lose weight, increase your rate of weight-loss and insure that lost pounds stay gone for good. Not only will exercise help you lose weight by burning more calories, but you'll also build muscle, which will help you burn more calories when you're at rest.

In addition, exercise has many other health benefits beyond weight loss. Research suggests that regular physical activity helps lower the risk of developing heart disease, Type 2 diabetes, high blood pressure, osteoporosis and certain forms of cancer. Numerous studies have found a strong inverse relationship between exercise and mortality from all causes in women. Specifically, exercise helps you feel better and improves health by:

- Lowering LDL (bad) cholesterol
- Raising HDL (good) cholesterol
- Lowering blood pressure
- Increasing your metabolic rate (which can help burn calories)
- Lowering blood sugar levels in Type 2 diabetes (and decreasing insulin resistance)
- Improving mood
- Decreasing stress levels
- Increasing energy levels

Best of all, you don't need to start training for a marathon in order to reap the benefits of exercise. All it takes are small changes in your exercise plan and daily activities. The chart below explains how the physical activities you do every day can add up over time.

Calories Burned During Daily Activities*			
ACTIVITY	TIME/CALORIES	FREQUENCY	CALORIES/FAT BURNED IN 3 MONTHS
Cleaning	60 min/300 calories	once a week	3,600/1 lb of fat
Cooking	30 min/108 calories	4x a week	5,184/1.5 lbs of fat
Gardening	60 min/420 calories	once a week	5,040/1.4 lbs of fat
Mowing the lawn	60 min/540 calories	once a week	6,480/1.9 lbs of fat
Washing the car	15 min/86 calories	once a week	1,032/0.3 lbs of fat
Washing windows	90 min/423 calories	4x a year	423/0.1 lbs of fat
Walking the dog	30 min/126 calories	Daily	10,584/3 lbs of fat

* Based on a woman who weighs 175 lbs.

WALK YOUR WAY FIT

WHEN IT COMES TO THE IDEAL EXERCISE, walking is pretty hard to beat. It's easy, low impact and requires no special equipment. There's plenty of research to show that regular brisk walking can help you lose weight just as easily as more strenuous exercise. Even better, walking is just as good as strenuous exercise at conferring a host of health benefits, including lower blood pressure, lower LDL (bad) cholesterol and higher HDL (good) cholesterol, and an improvement in insulin sensitivity. Since walking is a weight-bearing exercise, it will also increase your bone density, which helps reduce the risk of osteoporosis. Best of all, you'll start reaping most of these benefits within the first two to three weeks of regular walking.

The Keys to a Successful Walking Routine

BEFORE YOUR WALK

- Get a good pair of walking shoes. Look for shoes that have good cushioning and bend easily through the ball of the foot, but are firm and supportive through the arch.

- Wear loose, comfortable clothing that's appropriate for the weather.

- Be safe. Try to choose a route that does not have automobile traffic. If that's not possible, make sure the road has a wide shoulder, and always walk against traffic so you can see approaching cars. If you'll be walking before dawn or after dark, wear reflective clothing, and carry a whistle for extra safety.

DURING YOUR WALK

- Drink plenty of water. Drink a glass or two before you start and carry a water bottle with you. Afterward, replenish lost fluids with another two or three glasses.

- Warm up by walking slowly for the first few minutes to allow your muscles to loosen up, which will help prevent injury.

A NOTE FOR BEGINNERS

If you're starting a new exercise routine, it's important to first get your doctor's approval. After that, you'll want to begin slowly, especially if you've been completely sedentary. Starting out too quickly will leave you sore, discouraged and more prone to injury. Depending on your fitness level, you may have to start with something as simple as a five-minute walk around the block. Slow but steady is the rule. Before you know it, you'll notice that exercise has become easier and you'll be able to gradually increase the duration of your walks.

USE THE RIGHT TECHNIQUE

- Walk tall, lifting your chest and shoulders. Contract your stomach muscles to flatten your lower back. Land on your heel and roll your foot from heel to toe, pushing off forcefully with your toe.

- To go faster, concentrate on taking shorter, quicker steps rather than lengthening your stride. For an extra speed boost, bend your elbows to 90 degrees and swing your hands from your waist to chest high, holding your arms in unclenched fists.

- Always cool down by walking slowly for five minutes at the end of your walk, which will allow your heart rate to slow down gradually and help prevent muscle soreness.

What's Your Target Heart Rate?

When it comes to walking for weight loss and good health, a stroll around the mall is not going to cut it. To really see results, you've got to get your pulse up to your target heart rate (THR). This figure is based on a percentage of your maximum heart rate: the greatest number of times your heart beats per minute, as estimated based on your age.

When your heart is beating at about 50 to 60 percent of maximum, you begin to experience basic health benefits. Take it up to 60 to 70 percent, and you enter the weight-loss zone. Anywhere from 70 to 85 percent is considered ideal for overall aerobic fitness. Based on these ranges, experts often refer to your target heart-rate zone as between 65 and 85 percent of your maximum heart rate.

TO FIND YOUR TARGET HEART RATE ZONE:

1 Estimate your maximum heart rate by subtracting your age from 220, or get it measured during a stress test, a good idea for women over 50.

2 Multiply your maximum rate by .65 for the low end of your target zone and by .85 for the high end.

For example, a 35-year-old woman's maximum heart rate is 185 beats per minute, and her target zone is between 120 and 157 beats per minute.

Even without taking your pulse, you can still keep tabs on how intensely you're exercising. The easiest way is to perform a talk test. You should be able to talk when you need to, but you shouldn't be able to carry on a nonstop conversation. You should be breaking a light sweat, but not gasping for air.

Follow the walking workout (see box, *right*), and after four weeks, con-

---

A ONE-MONTH WALKING WORKOUT

WEEK 1: Walk for 20 minutes 2 times this week

WEEK 2: Walk for 20 minutes 3 times this week

WEEK 3: Walk for 30 minutes 3 times this week

WEEK 4: Walk for 35 to 40 minutes 3 to 4 times this week

tinue on the Week 4 schedule. Gradually work your way up to walking for 60 minutes at least four times a week.

- The plan above is geared toward beginning exercisers. If you've been walking fairly regularly, you may want to start with Week 3 or Week 4, and gradually work your way up to walking for 60 minutes, five or six times a week.

- If you can't find the time to fit in 30 to 45 minutes of walking all at one time, you can take three shorter walks over the course of the day. For instance, take a 20-minute walk before breakfast, a 25-minute walk on your lunch hour and a 15-minute walk after dinner.

- Once you've been walking for a few weeks, try integrating short bursts of speed into your routine. Every 10 minutes, pick a landmark in the near distance, such as a street sign, and quicken your pace until you reach it. These short bursts of intense walking with help keep your target heart rate high enough for optimal fat burning.

- Want an even more challenging workout? Add an area with more hills to your walking route. Or take a walk in the sand or go hiking. Walking on uneven terrain adds resistance to your workout, which makes it a tougher calorie burner.

Strength Training Matters

Do you ever wonder why men can get away with eating so many more calories than women without gaining as much weight, even at comparable body weights? The answer is because they're genetically programmed to have more muscle and less body fat. So if you want to optimize your body's fat-burning potential, you've got to make muscle-strengthening exercises a part of your exercise regimen.

Many women mistakenly believe that strength training will bulk them up and interfere with weight loss. Nothing could be further from the truth. Strength training will make you look fit, not bulky. Muscle is denser and tighter than fat, so transforming fat into muscle will "shrink" you in size. Muscle is much more energy-needy than fat so the more muscle mass you have, the more calories you burn at rest. By increasing your muscle mass by 3 pounds you will burn about 120 more calories each day, or about 840 calories each week.

By changing fat to muscle, you'll lose inches as well as pounds—and you'll burn calories at a higher rate every day. You don't need to spend hours at a health club or invest in expensive equipment. Many effective strength-training exercises use nothing more than your body's own resistance.

Here are some tips on starting a strength-training regimen:

- To ensure proper form, get some type of expert instruction. A few sessions with a trainer is ideal, but a video can also help you practice proper technique. This will help you avoid unnecessary injury.

- Strength train 2 or 3 times a week, with at least one rest day in between. Be mindful that you want to strengthen, not strain, muscles.

- The most effective resistance floor exercises are abdominal crunches, push-ups, leg lifts and squats.

- If you choose free weights, begin with 2- to 3-pound weights. You can buy a set of hand weights for about $10 at a sports equipment store. Or make your own out of empty 1-liter plastic soda bottles: Just fill them with water or sand and weigh them on a scale. Eventually you can work up to 5-pound weights.

- Do a variety of exercises for total body conditioning. Include exercises for the arms, shoulders, abdomen, back, chest, buttocks and legs.

- After you've been strength training for a few weeks, you can up the intensity of your workout by using heavier weights, doing more repetitions of each exercise or increasing the total number of exercises you do for each of the major muscle groups.

Here is a program for strength training your muscles. It is for women who are just beginning to strength train:

WEEK	REPETITIONS PER MUSCLE GROUP	SETS*	TOTAL TIME SPENT TRAINING ALL MUSCLES	FREQUENCY
1 & 2	12	2	15 minutes	2x a week
3 & 4	12	2–3	20 minutes	2–3x a week

* Each set represents a group of repetitions (12, for example) of the same movement. Therefore, two sets would give you a total of 24 repetitions. Be sure to rest a few moments between sets to avoid muscle fatigue.

In an Exercise Rut? How to Stay Motivated

Changing habits to transform a sedentary lifestyle into an active one is challenging, but the physical and mental benefits are phenomenal. If you want to live longer, feel better, be healthier and stay trimmer, you've got to be physically active. Consider the following to make exercise more interesting:

FIND A WALKING BUDDY. You'll be a lot less likely to hit the snooze button in the morning if you know someone will be waiting for you.

MIX IT UP. Vary the lengths of your walks, the routes and the times of day.

SET A PERFORMANCE GOAL. Plan to walk in a fundraiser or schedule a hiking vacation.

KEEP AN EXERCISE LOG. Seeing your progress on paper is very encouraging and a great way to stay motivated. There is a sample exercise log on page 160.

DO SOMETHING YOU REALLY ENJOY WHILE EXERCISING. Listen to your favorite music while strength training at home. Catch up on the news while walking on the treadmill.

TRY A GADGET. A pedometer is a great motivational tool. This beeper-size electronic device clips onto your waistband and measures the number of steps you take. Some models also keep track of your mileage and estimate the number of calories you've burned. These devices, which cost around $25 to $30, can be found at sporting goods stores.

ADD SOME ADVENTURE TO YOUR WORKOUT. Try a new sport or activity such as rock climbing, karate, kickboxing, yoga or Pilates.

7. The Woman's Day Plan for Weight Loss

30 SAMPLE MENUS

THE FOLLOWING MENUS WERE PREPARED TO GUIDE YOU in designing your daily meals, to illustrate how to count your food in terms of food exchanges and to offer you variety while following this weight-loss plan. Using these daily menus can make things easier for you, especially when you first begin the plan. Let the menus be a helpful guide, but don't allow them to restrict you. If you like to eat the same breakfast each day, that's fine—go ahead and eat cottage cheese and fruit every morning. If you don't like some of the food items on the sample menus, don't force yourself to eat them. Instead, substitute the foods you enjoy from the food choice lists (preferably from the best choice category).

As I've mentioned, weight loss is faster, and hunger diminished, when you eat meals low on the glycemic index (GI). There's an emphasis on keeping the GI of the meals in these menus low, too. However, you will see that the sample menus occasionally include foods that have a high GI: white-flour carbohydrates or a whole-wheat bagel. This is not an oversight on my part. You can make the change from a high glycemic way of eating to a diet rich in low GI foods and still enjoy small amounts of high GI foods from time to time. The goal is to limit these high glycemic foods, not to totally exclude them (unless you prefer to). This way you can lose weight successfully without feeling severely deprived.

Each sample day provides 1,200 calories with the recommended amounts of dietary fiber (20 to 35 g per day) and at least 1,000 mg of calcium. Each sample day gets 28 percent of its calories from protein, 27 percent from fat and 45 percent from carbohydrate. Bon appétit!

DAY 1

BREAKFAST	
½ cup fat-free or 1% fat cottage cheese	2 proteins
topped with sprinkle of cinnamon	free
and 4 walnut halves	1 fat
1 pear	1 fruit
Coffee or tea	free

LUNCH	
Turkey Sandwich:	
2 oz turkey breast	2 proteins
2 slices light rye toast	1 bread/starch
mustard/lettuce/tomato	free
1 dill pickle	free
1 cup salad greens	1 vegetable
1 Tbsp vinaigrette dressing	1 fat
Water or noncaloric beverage	free

AFTERNOON SNACK	
1 oz part-skim mozzarella cheese	1 protein
4 reduced-fat, weave-type crackers	1 bread/starch
2 clementines	1 fruit

DINNER	
1 medium baked chicken breast	
(3 oz edible portion)	3 proteins
1 medium (6 oz) sweet potato	2 bread/starches
1 cup steamed broccoli	2 vegetables
1 cup salad greens	1 vegetable
1 Tbsp vinaigrette dressing	1 fat
8 oz nonfat milk	1 dairy

EVENING SNACK	
8 oz nonfat plain or artificially sweetened yogurt	1 dairy
1 Tbsp chopped nuts	1 fat

DAY 2

BREAKFAST	
¾ cup of bran-flake cereal	1 bread/starch
1 small banana	1 fruit
8 oz nonfat milk	1 dairy
Coffee or tea	free

LUNCH	
Tuna in a Pita Pocket:	
3 oz water-packed tuna	3 proteins
1 Tbsp light mayonnaise	1 fat
1 Tbsp chopped celery	free
1 mini whole-wheat pita pocket	1 bread/starch
1 cup salad greens	1 vegetable
1 Tbsp vinaigrette dressing	1 fat
Water or noncaloric beverage	free

AFTERNOON SNACK	
1 apple	1 fruit
2 oz reduced-fat Cheddar cheese	2 proteins

DINNER	
3 oz London broil	3 proteins
⅓ cup cooked pearl barley	1 bread/starch
1 cup mixed vegetables	2 vegetables
1 cup salad greens	1 vegetable
1 Tbsp vinaigrette dressing	1 fat
Water or noncaloric beverage	free

EVENING SNACK	
8 oz nonfat milk	1 dairy
3 graham cracker squares	1 bread/starch
2 tsp natural peanut butter	1 fat

DAY 3

BREAKFAST

2 slices whole-grain pumpernickel toast	2 bread/starches
2 oz reduced-fat Swiss cheese	2 proteins
4 oz tomato juice	1 vegetable
Coffee or tea	free

LUNCH

Ham Sandwich:	
2 oz lean ham	2 proteins
lettuce/tomato/mustard	free
2 slices light rye bread	1 bread/starch
1 cup salad greens	1 vegetable
1 Tbsp vinaigrette dressing	1 fat
8 oz nonfat milk	1 dairy

AFTERNOON SNACK

¼ cup fat-free or 1% fat cottage cheese	1 protein
6 whole cashews	1 fat
1 pear	1 fruit

DINNER

3 oz broiled codfish	3 proteins
½ cup cooked bulgur wheat*	1 bread/starch
topped with 1 Tbsp chopped nuts	1 fat
1 cup steamed green beans	2 vegetables
1 cup salad greens	1 vegetable
1 Tbsp vinaigrette dressing	1 fat
Water or noncaloric beverage	free

EVENING SNACK

Yogurt Shake:	
4 oz nonfat milk	½ dairy
4 oz artificially sweetened peach yogurt	½ dairy
1 small banana	1 fruit
1 tsp vanilla extract	free
(Mix together in blender.)	

*Available at health food stores.

DAY 4

BREAKFAST

8 oz nonfat plain or artificially sweetened yogurt	1 dairy
1½ Tbsp trail mix	1 fat
1 apple	1 fruit
Coffee or tea	free

LUNCH

Roast Beef Sandwich:	
4 oz lean roast beef	4 proteins
mustard/lettuce/tomato	free
2 slices light rye toast	1 bread/starch
1 dill pickle	free
1 cup salad greens	1 vegetable
1 Tbsp vinaigrette dressing	1 fat
Water or noncaloric beverage	free

AFTERNOON SNACK

1 cup raw vegetable strips	1 vcgctablc
2 oz reduced-fat Cheddar cheese	2 protein
15 grapes	1 fruit

DINNER

Pasta Primavera:	
1 cup cooked bow-tie pasta	2 bread/starches
½ cup steamed broccoli	1 vegetable
½ cup steamed cauliflower	1 vegetable
2 oz part-skim mozzarella cheese in chunks	2 proteins
⅓ cup marinara sauce	1 vegetable
topped with 2 tsp Parmesan cheese	1 fat
1 cup salad greens	1 vegetable
1 Tbsp vinaigrette dressing	1 fat
Water or noncaloric beverage	free

EVENING SNACK

2 fig bars (½ oz *each*)	1 bread/starch
8 oz nonfat milk	1 dairy

DAY 5

BREAKFAST	
½ cup cooked oatmeal	1 bread/starch
topped with 1 Tbsp ground flaxseeds*	1 fat
½ grapefruit	1 fruit
Coffee or tea	free

LUNCH	
Salad Bar:	
2 cups fresh spinach leaves	2 vegetables
½ cup canned white beans	1 protein,
	1 bread/starch
1 Tbsp sunflower seeds	1 fat
2 oz shredded chicken breast	2 proteins
1 oz shredded reduced-fat cheese	1 protein
1 Tbsp vinaigrette dressing	1 fat
4 slices whole-wheat melba toast	1 bread/starch
Water or noncaloric beverage	free

AFTERNOON SNACK	
8 oz nonfat plain or artificially sweetened yogurt	1 dairy
1 apple	1 fruit

DINNER	
1 turkey breast (4 oz)	4 proteins
½ cup egg noodles	1 bread/starch
1 cup steamed zucchini and red peppers	2 vegetables
1 cup salad greens	1 vegetable
1 Tbsp vinaigrette dressing	1 fat
Water or noncaloric beverage	free

EVENING SNACK	
8 oz nonfat milk	1 dairy
½ cup sugar-free gelatin	free
1 Tbsp fat-free nondairy whipped topping	free

*Available at health food stores (buy whole, keep in refrigerator and grind before use).

DAY 6

BREAKFAST

½ pumpernickel bagel (2 oz)	2 bread/starches
1 Tbsp cream cheese	1 fat
1 tangerine	1 fruit
Coffee or tea	free

LUNCH

1 cup ready-to-use black bean soup	1 protein,
topped with 1 oz shredded	1 bread/starch
reduced-fat Swiss cheese	1 protein
2 sesame flatbreads (6 ½ in. by 1½ in.)	1 bread/starch
1 cup salad greens	1 vegetable
1 Tbsp vinaigrette dressing	1 fat
Water or noncaloric beverage	free

AFTERNOON SNACK

1 pear	1 fruit
4 walnut halves	1 fat

DINNER

1 large broiled chicken breast	
(6 oz edible portion)	6 proteins
1 cup steamed green beans	2 vegetables
topped with 1 Tbsp toasted almonds	1 fat
1 cup salad greens	1 vegetable
1 Tbsp fat-free salad dressing	free
8 oz nonfat milk	1 dairy

EVENING SNACK

8 oz nonfat plain or artificially sweetened yogurt	1 dairy

DAY 7

BREAKFAST

Low-Cholesterol Scrambled Eggs:	
4 egg whites or	
1 whole egg and 2 whites	2 proteins
½ cup chopped vegetables	1 vegetable
(Cook using nonstick cooking spray.)	
1 slice bacon	1 fat
Lettuce and tomato slices	free
4 oz vegetable juice	1 vegetable
Coffee or tea	free

LUNCH

1 vegetarian burger	1 protein, 1 bread/starch
in 1 mini whole-wheat pita pocket	1 bread/starch
with tomato/lettuce/onion/ketchup	free
1 cup salad greens	1 vegetable
½ Tbsp vinaigrette dressing	½ fat
1 apple	1 fruit
8 oz nonfat milk	1 dairy

AFTERNOON SNACK

10 baked tortilla chips	1 bread/starch
2 Tbsp tomato salsa	free

DINNER

1 serving Broiled Salmon with Olive Salsa*	4 proteins, 1 fat
¾ cup Wild Rice with Mushrooms and Red Pepper*	1 bread/starch, ½ fat
1 cup steamed spinach	2 vegetables
1 cup salad greens	1 vegetable
1 Tbsp vinaigrette dressing	1 fat
8 oz nonfat milk	1 dairy

EVENING SNACK

1 oz part-skim mozzarella cheese	1 protein
15 grapes	1 fruit

* Recipes included, pages 136 and 140.

DAY 8

BREAKFAST	
½ cup Wheatena-type cooked cereal	1 bread/starch
topped with 1 Tbsp ground flaxseeds*	1 fat
1 small banana	1 fruit
Coffee or tea	free

LUNCH	
Ham and Cheese Sandwich:	
3 oz lean ham	3 proteins
2 oz reduced-fat Swiss cheese	2 proteins
tomato/lettuce/mustard	free
2 slices light rye bread	1 bread/starch
1 dill pickle	free
1 cup salad greens	1 vegetable
1 Tbsp vinaigrette dressing	1 fat
Water or noncaloric beverage	free

AFTERNOON SNACK	
8 oz nonfat plain or artificially sweetened yogurt	1 dairy
1 pear	1 fruit

DINNER	
Chinese Takeout:	
1½ cups shrimp and Chinese vegetables	3 proteins,
	2 vegetables,
	2 fats
⅔ cup brown rice	2 bread/starches
1 cup salad greens	1 vegetable
1 Tbsp fat-free salad dressing	free
1 fortune cookie	free
Water or noncaloric beverage	free

EVENING SNACK	
½ cup sugar-free, fat-free butterscotch pudding**	1 dairy
1 Tbsp fat-free nondairy whipped topping	free

*Available at health food stores (buy whole, keep in refrigerator and grind before use).
**Available as a mix at the supermarket.

DAY 9

BREAKFAST	
½ whole-wheat bagel (2 oz)	2 bread/starches
1 Tbsp cream cheese	1 fat
½ grapefruit	1 fruit
Coffee or tea	free

LUNCH	
Corned Beef Sandwich:	
3 oz lean corned beef	3 proteins
lettuce/tomato/mustard	free
2 slices light rye toast	1 bread/starch
1 dill pickle	free
1 cup salad greens	1 vegetable
1 Tbsp vinaigrette dressing	1 fat
Water or noncaloric beverage	free

AFTERNOON SNACK	
8 oz nonfat plain or artificially sweetened yogurt	1 dairy
6 whole almonds	1 fat

DINNER	
4 oz baked scrod	4 proteins
½ cup ziti pasta	1 bread/starch
topped with 1 oz part-skim mozzarella	
cheese in chunks	1 protein
¼ cup marinara sauce	free
1 cup steamed broccoli	2 vegetables
1 cup salad greens	1 vegetable
1 Tbsp vinaigrette dressing	1 fat
Water or noncaloric beverage	free

EVENING SNACK	
8 oz nonfat milk	1 dairy
1 small banana	1 fruit

DAY 10

BREAKFAST

½ cup fat-free or 1% fat cottage cheese	2 proteins
topped with sprinkle of cinnamon	free
and 4 walnut halves	1 fat
1 apple	1 fruit
8 oz nonfat milk	1 dairy
Coffee or tea	free

LUNCH

Turkey Sandwich:	
3 oz turkey breast	3 proteins
tomato/lettuce	free
1 Tbsp light mayonnaise	1 fat
2 slices light whole-wheat bread	1 bread/starch
1 cup salad greens	1 vegetable
1 Tbsp vinaigrette dressing	1 fat
8 oz nonfat milk	1 dairy

AFTERNOON SNACK

1 cup raw vegetable strips	1 vegetable
4 oz tomato juice	1 vegetable

DINNER

12 mini cheese-filled ravioli	3 bread/starches,
(1½-in.-square ravioli)	2 proteins
⅓ cup marinara sauce	1 vegetable
1 cup salad greens	1 vegetable
1 Tbsp vinaigrette dressing	1 fat
1 cup steamed green beans	2 vegetables
Water or noncaloric beverage	free

EVENING SNACK

1 pear	1 fruit
1 oz reduced-fat Cheddar cheese	1 protein

DAY 11

BREAKFAST

¾ cup multigrain cereal*	1 bread/starch
8 oz nonfat milk	1 dairy
1 cup berries	1 fruit
Coffee or tea	free

LUNCH

Salmon Salad:	
2 cups salad greens	2 vegetables
4 oz canned salmon**	4 proteins
10 green olives	1 fat
1 Tbsp fat-free salad dressing	free
2 medium breadsticks	1 bread/starch
Water or noncaloric beverage	free

AFTERNOON SNACK

6 whole cashews	1 fat
2 clementines	1 fruit

DINNER

1 turkey burger (4 oz)	4 proteins
½ cup corn	1 bread/starch
1 cup cooked spinach	2 vegetables
1 cup salad greens	1 vegetable
1 Tbsp vinaigrette dressing	1 fat
Water or noncaloric beverage	free

EVENING SNACK

3 Healthy Chocolate Chip Cookies†	1 bread/starch, 1 fat
8 oz nonfat milk	1 dairy

* Look for cereal with 5 g (or more) dietary fiber per serving.
** Good source of calcium (tiny bones are edible).
† Recipe included, page 145.

DAY 12

BREAKFAST

1 whole-wheat English muffin	2 bread/starches
1 Tbsp trans-fat-free diet margarine	1 fat
1 cup melon cubes	1 fruit
8 oz nonfat milk	1 dairy
Coffee or tea	free

LUNCH

Tuna in a Pita Pocket:

3 oz water-packed tuna	3 proteins
1 Tbsp light mayonnaise	1 fat
1 Tbsp chopped celery	free
1 mini whole-wheat pita pocket	1 bread/starch
1 cup salad greens	1 vegetable
1 Tbsp fat-free salad dressing	free
Water or noncaloric beverage	free

AFTERNOON SNACK

1 apple	1 fruit
1 oz part-skim mozzarella cheese	1 protein

DINNER

1 medium broiled center-cut pork chop (4 oz edible portion)	4 proteins
1 cup steamed red cabbage	2 vegetables
1 serving Tasty Bulgur with Olives and Peppers*	1 bread/starch, 1 fat
1 cup salad greens	1 vegetable
1 Tbsp vinaigrette dressing	1 fat
Water or noncaloric beverage	free

EVENING SNACK

8 oz nonfat plain or artificially sweetened yogurt	1 dairy

* Recipe included, page 144.

DAY 13

BREAKFAST	
1 hard-boiled egg, or 2 hard-boiled egg whites	1 protein
1 sausage link	1 fat
1 slice light whole-wheat toast	½ bread/starch
½ grapefruit	1 fruit
8 oz nonfat milk	1 dairy
Coffee or tea	free

LUNCH	
1 slice pizzeria cheese pizza	2 bread/starches, 2 proteins, 2 fats, 1 vegetable
2 cups salad greens	2 vegetables
1 Tbsp fat-free salad dressing	free
Water or noncaloric beverage	free

AFTERNOON SNACK	
1½ Tbsp hummus*	1 fat
2 reduced-fat, weave-type crackers	½ bread/starch
15 grapes	1 fruit

DINNER	
1 boneless, skinless chicken breast (4 oz edible portion) (Coat with 2 Tbsp barbecue sauce and broil.)	4 proteins
⅓ cup brown rice	1 bread/starch
1 cup mixed vegetables	2 vegetables
topped with 1 oz shredded reduced-fat Swiss cheese	1 protein
1 cup salad greens	1 vegetable
1 Tbsp fat-free salad dressing	free
Water or noncaloric beverage	free

EVENING SNACK	
½ cup sugar-free, fat-free vanilla pudding**	1 dairy

* Ready-to-use hummus or recipe on page 134.
** Available as a mix at the supermarket.

DAY 14

BREAKFAST	
2 slices light rye toast	1 bread/starch
2 oz reduced-fat Cheddar cheese	2 proteins
1 tangerine	1 fruit
8 oz nonfat milk	1 dairy
Coffee or tea	free

LUNCH	
8 oz ready-to-use lentil soup	1 protein, 1 bread/starch
2 cups salad greens	2 vegetables
1 Tbsp vinaigrette dressing	1 fat
Water or noncaloric beverage	free

AFTERNOON SNACK	
4 oz nonfat plain or artificially sweetened yogurt	½ dairy
1½ Tbsp trail mix	1 fat

DINNER	
2 medium broiled lamb chops (5 oz edible portion)	5 proteins
1 medium (6 oz) sweet potato	2 bread/starches
1 cup steamed cauliflower	2 vegetables
1 cup salad greens	1 vegetable
1 Tbsp vinaigrette dressing	1 fat
Water or noncaloric beverage	free

EVENING SNACK	
1 serving Apple and Pear Parfait*	½ dairy, 1 fruit, 1 fat

* Recipe included, page 146.

DAY 15

BREAKFAST

2 slices raisin bread	2 bread/starches
½ Tbsp cream cheese	½ fat
Coffee or tea	free

LUNCH

Fast Food Taco Lunch:

2 medium tacos filled with ground beef, shredded lettuce and cheese	2 bread/starches, 2 proteins, 2½ fats
taco sauce	free
1 cup salad greens	1 vegetable
1 Tbsp fat-free salad dressing	free
Water or noncaloric beverage	free

AFTERNOON SNACK

8 oz nonfat plain or artificially sweetened yogurt	1 dairy

DINNER

1 baked chicken breast (6 oz, skinless)	6 proteins
1 cup steamed green beans	2 vegetables
1 cup salad greens	1 vegetable
1 Tbsp fat-free salad dressing	free
Water or noncaloric beverage	free

EVENING SNACK

1 serving Mocha Float*	1 dairy, 2 fruits, 1 fat

* Recipe included, page 146.

DAY 16

BREAKFAST	
¾ cup high-fiber 7-grain twigs and sesame cereal*	1 bread/starch
8 oz nonfat milk	1 dairy
1 peach	1 fruit
Coffee or tea	free

LUNCH	
8 oz nonfat plain or artificially sweetened yogurt	1 dairy
1½ Tbsp trail mix	1 fat
2 sesame flatbreads (6½ in. by 1½ in.)	1 bread/starch
1 cup salad greens	1 vegetable
1 Tbsp vinaigrette dressing	1 fat
Water or noncaloric beverage	free

AFTERNOON SNACK	
1 apple, sliced,	1 fruit
with 2 tsp natural peanut butter	1 fat

DINNER	
1 grilled hamburger (6 oz, made from extra-lean ground beef)	6 proteins
1 serving Cold Bean Salad**	1 bread/starch, 1 protein, 1 fat
2 cups salad greens	2 vegetables
2 Tbsp fat-free salad dressing	free
Water or noncaloric beverage	free

EVENING SNACK	
1 oz reduced-fat Cheddar cheese	1 protein
1 cup raw vegetable sticks	1 vegetable
4 reduced-fat, weave-type crackers	1 bread/starch

* Available at most health food stores. Provides 8 to 10 g dietary fiber per serving.
** Recipe included, page 142.

DAY 17

BREAKFAST

¾ cup bran-flake cereal	1 bread/starch
8 oz nonfat milk	1 dairy
1 small banana	1 fruit
Coffee or tea	free

LUNCH

Roast Beef Sandwich:	
2 oz roast beef	2 proteins
2 slices light rye toast	1 bread/starch
mustard/tomato	free
1 pickle	free
1 cup salad greens	1 vegetable
1 Tbsp vinaigrette dressing	1 fat
1 apple	1 fruit
Water or noncaloric beverage	free

AFTERNOON SNACK

2 oz reduced-fat Cheddar cheese	2 proteins
4 reduced-fat, weave-type crackers	1 bread/starch

DINNER

1 serving Apricot-Lemon Glazed Fish Fillet*	4 proteins
1 cup steamed broccoli	2 vegetables
⅓ cup pearl barley	1 bread/starch
2 cups salad greens	2 vegetables
2 Tbsp vinaigrette dressing	2 fats
Water or noncaloric beverage	free

EVENING SNACK

8 oz nonfat plain or artificially sweetened yogurt with 6 whole cashews	1 dairy 1 fat

* Recipe included, page 136.

DAY 18

BREAKFAST

Reduced-Fat Omelet:	
1 whole egg and 2 egg whites or 4 egg whites	2 proteins
½ cup total chopped onion, peppers and tomatoes	1 vegetable
(Cook in 1 tsp olive oil.)	1 fat
1 cup melon cubes	1 fruit
8 oz nonfat milk	1 dairy
Coffee or tea	free

LUNCH

1 vegetarian burger, grilled	1 protein, 1 bread/starch
with 1 oz reduced-fat American cheese	1 protein
on 1 mini whole-wheat pita pocket	1 bread/starch
with onion/ketchup/tomato	free
1 cup salad greens	1 vegetable
1 Tbsp vinaigrette dressing	1 fat
1 pear	1 fruit
Water or noncaloric beverage	free

AFTERNOON SNACK

8 oz nonfat plain or artificially sweetened yogurt	1 dairy

DINNER

1 turkey breast (4 oz)	4 proteins
½ medium baked sweet potato (3 oz)	1 bread/starch
1 cup grilled zucchini and red peppers	1 vegetable
(Brush with 1 tsp olive oil before grilling.)	1 fat
1 cup salad greens	1 vegetable
1 Tbsp vinaigrette dressing	1 fat
Water or noncaloric beverage	free

EVENING SNACK

3 cups hot-air-popped or microwave light popcorn	1 bread/starch

DAY 19

BREAKFAST

¾ cup Wheatena-type hot cereal	1 bread/starch
with 1 Tbsp chopped walnuts	1 fat
and dash of cinnamon	free
1 nectarine	1 fruit
Coffee or tea	free

LUNCH

Salad with Turkey Strips:	
2 cups salad greens	2 vegetables
4 oz turkey strips	4 proteins
1 oz shredded reduced-fat cheese	1 protein
1 Tbsp vinaigrette dressing	1 fat
8 oz nonfat milk	1 dairy

AFTERNOON SNACK

1 oz reduced-fat Swiss cheese	1 protein
1 pear	1 fruit

DINNER

Pasta Primavera:	
1 cup cooked ziti pasta	2 bread/starches
1 cup mixed vegetables	2 vegetables
⅓ cup marinara sauce	1 vegetable
2 oz part-skim mozzarella cheese in chunks	2 proteins
2 cups salad greens	2 vegetables
1 Tbsp vinaigrette dressing	1 fat
Water or noncaloric beverage	free

EVENING SNACK

3 graham cracker squares	1 bread/starch
2 tsp natural peanut butter	1 fat
8 oz nonfat milk	1 dairy

DAY 20

BREAKFAST	
1 whole-wheat English muffin	2 bread/starches
1 Tbsp trans-fat-free diet margarine	1 fat
1 cup melon cubes	1 fruit
Coffee or tea	free

LUNCH	
Tuna Salad and Cheese Sandwich:	
2 slices light whole-wheat bread	1 bread/starch
3 oz white tuna, water-packed	3 proteins
1 Tbsp light mayonnaise	1 fat
2 Tbsp chopped onion	free
1 oz reduced-fat Swiss cheese	1 protein
1 cup salad greens	1 vegetable
1 Tbsp fat-free salad dressing	free
½ pear, sliced	½ fruit
8 oz nonfat milk	1 dairy

AFTERNOON SNACK	
½ cup frozen yogurt	1 bread/starch
with 1½ Tbsp trail mix	1 fat

DINNER	
1 serving Pan-Fried Pork Chops with Fruit Chutney*	4 proteins
	½ fruit
1 cup steamed zucchini	2 vegetables
1 cup salad greens	1 vegetable
1 Tbsp fat-free salad dressing	free
Water or noncaloric beverage	free

EVENING SNACK	
8 oz nonfat plain or artificially sweetened yogurt	1 dairy
top with 4 walnut halves	1 fat

* Recipe included, page 135.

DAY 21

BREAKFAST	
1 slice Yogurt, Lemon and	1 bread/starch,
Poppy Seed Bread, toasted*	½ fat
½ Tbsp trans-fat-free diet margarine	½ fat
1 cup berries	1 fruit
8 oz nonfat milk	1 dairy
Coffee or tea	free

LUNCH	
Ham and Cheese Sandwich:	
2 oz ham	2 proteins
2 oz reduced-fat Swiss cheese	2 proteins
tomato/lettuce/mustard	free
2 slices light rye toast	1 bread/starch
1 cup salad greens	1 vegetable
1 Tbsp vinaigrette dressing	1 fat
8 oz nonfat milk	1 dairy

AFTERNOON SNACK	
3 graham cracker squares	1 bread/starch
2 tsp peanut butter	1 fat

DINNER	
Restaurant Meal:	
1 glass white wine	1 bread/starch
4 oz grilled shrimp	4 proteins
1 cup steamed mixed vegetables	2 vegetables
1 cup salad greens	1 vegetable
1 Tbsp vinaigrette dressing	1 fat
1 cup melon cubes	1 fruit
Water or noncaloric beverage	free

EVENING SNACK	
½ cup sugar-free gelatin	free
with 1 Tbsp fat-free nondairy whipped topping	free

* Recipe included, page 145.

DAY 22

BREAKFAST	
1 serving Breakfast Smoothie*	1 dairy, 1 fruit 1 fat
Coffee or tea	free
LUNCH	
1 serving Feta Cheese Wrap*	1½ protein, 2 bread/starches, 2 vegetables, 2 fats
½ apple	½ fruit
Water or noncaloric beverage	free
AFTERNOON SNACK	
1 oz reduced-fat Cheddar cheese	1 protein
½ cup berries	½ fruit
DINNER	
1 boneless, skinless chicken breast (5½ oz)	5½ proteins
½ medium sweet potato (3 oz)	1 bread/starch
1 cup steamed green beans	2 vegetables
1 cup salad greens	1 vegetable
1 Tbsp vinaigrette dressing	1 fat
Water or noncaloric beverage	free
EVENING SNACK	
2 fig bars	1 bread/starch
8 oz nonfat milk	1 dairy

* Recipes included, pages 132 and 139.

DAY 23

BREAKFAST

8 oz nonfat plain or artificially sweetened yogurt	1 dairy
topped with sprinkle of cinnamon	free
and 4 walnut halves	1 fat
1 pear, sliced	1 fruit
Coffee or tea	free

LUNCH

Corned Beef Sandwich:	
4 oz lean corned beef	4 proteins
lettuce/tomato/mustard	free
2 slices light rye toast	1 bread/starch
1 dill pickle	free
1 cup salad greens	1 vegetable
1 Tbsp vinaigrette dressing	1 fat
Water or noncaloric beverage	free

AFTERNOON SNACK

8 oz nonfat milk	1 dairy
1 apple	1 fruit
10 peanuts	1 fat

DINNER

1 serving Vegetarian Chili*	3 bread/starches, 2 vegetables, 1 protein
topped with 1 oz shredded reduced-fat Swiss cheese	1 protein
1 cup salad greens	1 vegetable
1 Tbsp vinaigrette dressing	1 fat
Water or noncaloric beverage	free

EVENING SNACK

2 oz reduced-fat Cheddar cheese	2 proteins

* Recipe included, page 137.

DAY 24

BREAKFAST

2 slices whole-grain pumpernickel toast	2 bread/starches
2 oz part-skim mozzarella cheese	2 proteins
½ grapefruit	1 fruit
Coffee or tea	free

LUNCH

Salad Bar:	
2 cups salad greens	2 vegetables
1 oz reduced-fat Cheddar cheese	1 protein
½ cup chickpeas (canned)	1 protein, 1 bread/starch
1½ Tbsp sunflower seeds	1½ fats
2 Tbsp fat-free salad dressing	free
Water or noncaloric beverage	free

AFTERNOON SNACK

8 oz nonfat plain or artificially sweetened yogurt	1 dairy
1 cup berries	1 fruit
6 cashews	1 fat

DINNER

1 serving of Chicken Vegetable Stir-Fry*	4 proteins, 2 vegetables, ½ fat
⅓ cup wild rice	1 bread/starch
1 cup salad greens	1 vegetable
1 Tbsp vinaigrette dressing	1 fat
Water or noncaloric beverage	free

EVENING SNACK

8 oz nonfat milk	1 dairy
½ cup sugar-free gelatin	free
with 1 Tbsp fat-free nondairy topping	free

* Recipe included, page 137.

DAY 25

BREAKFAST	
½ whole-wheat bagel (2 oz)	2 bread/starches
1 Tbsp cream cheese	1 fat
8 oz nonfat milk	1 dairy
Coffee or tea	free
LUNCH	
½ cup fat-free or 1% fat cottage cheese	2 proteins
topped with 6 whole almonds	1 fat
1 peach	1 fruit
1 cup salad greens	1 vegetable
1 Tbsp vinaigrette dressing	1 fat
Water or noncaloric beverage	free
AFTERNOON SNACK	
Cheesy Popcorn:	
3 cups hot-air-popped or microwave light popcorn	1 bread/starch
(Toss with 1 oz shredded part-skim mozzarella cheese.)	1 protein
DINNER	
1 grilled hamburger (5 oz)	5 proteins
in a mini whole-wheat pita pocket	1 bread/starch
with ketchup/onion	free
1 cup steamed broccoli	2 vegetables
1 cup salad greens	1 vegetable
1 Tbsp vinaigrette dressing	1 fat
Water or noncaloric beverage	free
EVENING SNACK	
8 oz nonfat milk	1 dairy
1 pear	1 fruit

DAY 26

BREAKFAST	
1 oat-bran English muffin	2 bread/starches
1 Tbsp trans-fat-free diet margarine	1 fat
1 orange	1 fruit
Coffee or tea	free

LUNCH	
1 cup ready-to-use lentil soup	1 protein, 1 bread/starch
2 cups salad greens	2 vegetables
1 Tbsp vinaigrette dressing	1 fat
1 apple	1 fruit
8 oz nonfat milk	1 dairy

AFTERNOON SNACK	
1 oz part-skim mozzarella cheese	1 protein
1 cup fresh vegetable strips	1 vegetable

DINNER	
1 broiled turkey burger (6 oz, made from ground turkey breast)	6 proteins
½ cup cooked bulgur wheat*	1 bread/starch
1 cup steamed baby carrots	2 vegetables
2 cups salad greens	2 vegetables
2 Tbsp vinaigrette dressing	2 fats
Water or noncaloric beverage	free

EVENING SNACK	
8 oz nonfat plain or artificially sweetened yogurt	1 dairy

*Available at health food stores.

DAY 27

BREAKFAST	
Low-Cholesterol Scrambled Eggs:	
1 whole egg and 2 egg whites, or 4 egg whites	2 proteins
(Cook in 1 tsp oil.)	1 fat
1 medium tomato, sliced	1 vegetable
1 slice 7-grain toast	1 bread/starch
Coffee or tea	free
LUNCH	
1 serving Pear and Chicken Salad*	3 proteins,
	1 bread/starch,
	2 vegetables,
	1 fruit,
	2 fats
8 oz nonfat milk	1 dairy
AFTERNOON SNACK	
1 serving Tomato, Basil and Barley Bisque*	1 bread/starch,
	½ dairy
DINNER	
1 small broiled pork chop (3 oz edible portion)	3 proteins
⅓ cup wild rice	1 bread/starch
1 cup steamed spinach	2 vegetables
1 cup salad greens	1 vegetable
1 Tbsp vinaigrette dressing	1 fat
Water or noncaloric beverage	free
EVENING SNACK	
4 oz nonfat plain or artificially sweetened yogurt	½ dairy
1 cup berries	1 fruit

* Recipes included, pages 138 and 134.

DAY 28

BREAKFAST	
2 slices light whole-wheat toast	1 bread/starch
1 Tbsp trans-fat-free diet margarine	1 fat
4 oz vegetable juice	1 vegetable
Coffee or tea	free

LUNCH	
Low-Fat Grilled Cheese Sandwich:	
2 oz reduced-fat American cheese	2 proteins
2 slices fresh tomato	free
2 slices light whole-wheat bread	1 bread/starch
1 Tbsp trans-fat-free diet margarine	1 fat
(Cook in nonstick skillet.)	
1 cup salad greens	1 vegetable
1 Tbsp vinaigrette dressing	1 fat
1 pear	1 fruit
8 oz nonfat milk	1 dairy

AFTERNOON SNACK	
½ cup fat-free or 1% fat cottage cheese	2 proteins
½ cup berries	½ fruit

DINNER	
4 oz roasted turkey breast	4 proteins,
with 1 serving Fruit Stuffing*	2 bread/starches,
	½ fruit
and 1 Tbsp gravy	free
1 cup steamed broccoli and cauliflower florets	2 vegetables
1 cup salad greens	1 vegetable
1 Tbsp vinaigrette dressing	1 fat
Water or noncaloric beverage	free

EVENING SNACK	
8 oz nonfat plain or artificially sweetened yogurt	1 dairy

* Recipe included, page 143.

DAY 29

BREAKFAST

½ cup fat-free or 1% fat cottage cheese	2 proteins
1 peach	1 fruit
4 slices whole-wheat melba toast	1 bread/starch
Coffee or tea	free

LUNCH

Turkey Sandwich:	
2 oz lean turkey	2 proteins
2 slices light whole-wheat toast	1 bread/starch
mustard/lettuce/tomato	free
1 cup salad greens	1 vegetable
1 Tbsp vinaigrette dressing	1 fat
Water or noncaloric beverage	free

AFTERNOON SNACK

8 oz nonfat plain or artificially sweetened yogurt	1 dairy
3 graham cracker squares	1 bread/starch

DINNER

4 oz broiled scrod	4 proteins
1 serving Sweet Potato Oven Fries*	1 bread/starch, 1 fat
1 serving Oven Roasted Vegetables*	1 vegetable, 1 fat
2 cups salad greens	2 vegetables
1 Tbsp vinaigrette dressing	1 fat
Water or noncaloric beverage	free

EVENING SNACK

8 oz nonfat milk	1 dairy
1 banana	1 fruit

* Recipes included, pages 141 and 142.

DAY 30

BREAKFAST

1 Cranberry-Nut Muffin*	1½ bread/starch, 1 fat
1 cup melon cubes	1 fruit
8 oz nonfat milk	1 dairy
Coffee or tea	free

LUNCH

Salad with Chicken Strips:

2 cups salad greens	2 vegetables
1 cup raw vegetable strips	1 vegetable
4 oz chicken strips	4 proteins
1 oz shredded reduced-fat cheese	1 protein
4 walnut halves	1 fat
1 Tbsp vinaigrette dressing	1 fat
8 oz nonfat milk	1 dairy

AFTERNOON SNACK

½ cup fat-free or 1% fat cottage cheese	2 proteins
½ peach, sliced	½ fruit

DINNER

1 serving Bow-Tie Pasta with Beans and Vegetables*	2½ bread/starches, 1 protein, 1 fat
1 cup salad greens	1 vegetable
1 Tbsp fat-free salad dressing	free
Water or noncaloric beverage	free

EVENING SNACK

1 serving Hot Spiced Apple-Cranberry Cider*	½ fruit

* Recipes included, pages 132, 138 and 133.

Breakfast Smoothie

8 oz (1 cup) nonfat plain yogurt
1 cup 1% lowfat or nonfat milk
1¼ cup whole fresh or frozen
    strawberries, hulled
1 fresh peach, peeled and sliced,
    or ¾ cup frozen peach slices (see Note)
2 tsp vanilla extract
2 Tbsp chopped walnuts
2 whole strawberries (optional)

1 Place first 5 ingredients in a blender. Purée mixture for 15 to 20 seconds.

2 Pour into two tall glasses and top each with 1 Tbsp chopped nuts.

3 Garnish glass with strawberry, if desired.

Note: If you prefer a thicker smoothie, replace the peach with 1 small sliced banana.

YIELD:	2 servings
SERVING SIZE:	10 oz
CALORIES:	207
COUNT AS:	1 dairy
	1 fruit
	1 fat

Start off your day right with a drink that provides a whopping 30 percent of your daily calcium needs.

Cranberry-Nut Muffins

1 cup nonfat milk
1 large egg
2 Tbsp olive oil
1 tsp vanilla extract
1 cup old-fashioned oats
¾ cup whole-wheat flour
¾ cup all-purpose flour
2 Tbsp sugar
1 Tbsp baking powder
¼ tsp salt
1 tsp ground cinnamon
1 cup fresh or frozen cranberries, chopped
TOPPING
    ¼ cup finely chopped walnuts
    1 Tbsp brown sugar
    1 Tbsp wheat germ

1 Heat oven to 400°F. Spray a 12-cup muffin pan with nonstick spray.

2 Whisk together first 4 ingredients. Stir in oats; set aside.

3 In a separate bowl, combine flours, sugar, baking powder, salt and cinnamon. Add milk mixture and stir until just blended. Fold in cranberries.

4 Fill muffin cups ⅔ full. Mix Topping ingredients and sprinkle on top of muffins. Bake 22 to 24 minutes or until a wooden pick inserted in centers comes out clean.

YIELD:	12 muffins
SERVING SIZE:	1 muffin
CALORIES:	145
COUNT AS:	1½ bread/starches
	1 fat

The oatmeal in this recipe contains water-soluble fiber, which is great for dieters because it absorbs water and expands in your stomach, making you feel full longer.

Hot Spiced Apple-Cranberry Cider

1 cup apple juice
1 cup cranberry-raspberry juice
1 Tbsp lemon juice
1 cup water
¼ tsp ground allspice
4 cinnamon sticks
4 apple slices, for garnish

1 Combine juices, water and ground all-spice in a medium saucepan.

2 Bring to a simmer over low heat, stirring to combine ingredients.

3 Pour into 4 teacups or mugs.

4 Serve with a cinnamon stick-stirrer and one fresh apple wedge, if desired

YIELD:	3 cups/4 servings
SERVING SIZE:	6 oz
CALORIES:	39
COUNT AS:	½ fruit

This drink, which can be served hot or cold, has only about half the calories of traditional hot apple cider.

Herb and Avocado Canapés

8 oz (1 cup) nonfat plain yogurt
1 Tbsp chopped scallion or onion
1 tsp lemon juice
1 tsp chopped fresh dill, plus fronds
   for garnish
4 slices whole-grain, high-fiber bread
   (with 3 g fiber per slice)
½ fresh avocado, thinly sliced (see Note)
2 small plum tomatoes, very thinly sliced
8 stuffed green olives, halved crosswise

1 To thicken the yogurt, place it in a paper towel–lined strainer set over a bowl or pan to collect the fluid. Let yogurt drain in the refrigerator for 1 to 3 hours. (The longer you allow the yogurt to drain, the thicker it becomes.)

2 In a bowl, stir together scallion, lemon juice, dill and thickened yogurt.

3 Toast the bread. Cut off the crusts, spread with yogurt mixture, then cut each slice into 4 squares.

4 Top each square with avocado and tomato slices. Place ½ green olive on top of each.

Note: To keep the avocado slices from browning, rinse them lightly with cool water after slicing.

YIELD:	4 servings
SERVING SIZE:	4 canapés
CALORIES:	145
COUNT AS:	1 bread/starch
	1 fat
	¼ dairy

Don't let a cocktail party invitation take a bite out of your dieting plans. Offer to bring this delicious, low-calorie appetizer.

Quick Hummus and Pitas

1 can (15 oz) chickpeas
   (garbanzo beans), drained and rinsed
1 garlic clove, crushed
2 Tbsp olive oil
2 Tbsp fresh lemon juice
½ tsp paprika
⅛ tsp cumin
2 to 4 Tbsp water
4 whole-wheat pita pockets
Garnish: parsley sprigs (optional)

1 Place beans and garlic in food processor and pulse to finely chop. Add oil, lemon juice, spices and 2 Tbsp water and process until smooth. Add up to 2 Tbsp more water if desired.

2 Transfer to covered container and chill for at least one hour or overnight.

3 Cut each pita into 6 triangles (24 total). Serve with the hummus.

YIELD:	1 cup/8 servings
SERVING SIZE:	2 Tbsp hummus and 3 pita triangles (½ pita)
CALORIES:	146
COUNT AS:	1 bread/starch 1½ fats

This spread measures very low on the glycemic index and is lower in fat than sour cream or guacamole.

Tomato, Basil and Barley Bisque

½ cup dry pearled barley
1 cup boiling water
2 tsp olive oil
1 yellow onion, chopped (about 1 cup)
2 cans (28 oz *each*) crushed tomatoes
4 cups nonfat milk
2 Tbsp all-purpose flour
⅓ cup chopped fresh basil
Salt and pepper

1 Rinse barley in cold water and place in small bowl. Add boiling water, cover and let stand for 30 minutes.

2 Heat oil in medium saucepan over medium-high heat. Add onion and cook, stirring, until golden, about 3 minutes.

3 Drain barley and add to pan along with tomatoes. Simmer over low heat for 30 minutes, stirring often.

4 In a separate medium saucepan, add 3¾ cups milk and heat slowly over low heat. Whisk the remaining ¼ cup milk with the flour. Add the flour mixture to the heated milk in the pan. Continue to heat slowly over low heat for 10 minutes, stirring occasionally. Do not bring to a boil.

5 Stir milk mixture into tomato/barley mixture. Stir in basil, season with salt and pepper to taste and serve.

YIELD:	10 servings
SERVING SIZE:	1 cup
CALORIES:	120
COUNT AS:	1 bread/starch ½ dairy

Cooked tomatoes are a great source of lycopene, an antioxidant that may help protect against heart disease and cancer.

The Kitchen Sink Vegetable Soup

2 tsp olive oil
1 large yellow onion, chopped
2 garlic cloves, chopped
8 cups water
2 to 4 chicken or vegetable bouillon cubes
2 cups small broccoli florets
2 cups baby carrots, sliced crosswise
1½ cups thinly sliced celery
1 cup green beans, rinsed and cut in half
2 medium bell peppers (1 red, 1 yellow), quartered lengthwise and thinly sliced crosswise
Salt and pepper

1 Heat oil in a large pot over medium-high heat. Add onion and garlic and cook, stirring, until golden, about 3 minutes.

2 Add water, bouillon cubes and vegetables and bring to a boil.

3 Simmer until vegetables are tender, about 30 minutes. Season with salt and pepper to taste.

YIELD:	10 servings
SERVING SIZE:	1 cup
CALORIES:	30
COUNT AS:	1 vegetable
	May be considered a free food

Studies show that eating soup as a first course helps curb your appetite so you eat a lighter second course.

Pan-Fried Pork Chops with Fruit Chutney

2 tsp olive oil
½ cup chopped onion
1 pear, cut in bite-size pieces
1 apple, cut in bite-size pieces
⅔ cup fresh or frozen cranberries
⅓ cup water
¼ teaspoon *each* garlic powder, salt and pepper
4 center-cut pork chops, about 1 in. thick (8 oz *each*)
Salt and pepper

1 Prepare fruit compote: Heat oil in medium saucepan over medium heat. Add onion and cook, stirring, for 2 minutes. Add pear, apple, cranberries and water. Reduce heat and simmer, stirring occasionally, 10 minutes, until fruit is tender and saucy.

2 Meanwhile sprinkle garlic powder, salt and pepper on both sides of pork chops.

3 Spray a large nonstick or cast-iron skillet with nonstick cooking spray and place over medium-high heat. Add chops and cook about 5 minutes per side, turning once. Transfer to plates and let stand for 5 minutes.

4 Season fruit mixture with salt and pepper and serve with the chops.

YIELD:	4 servings
SERVING SIZE:	1 pork chop with ⅓ cup chutney topping
CALORIES:	203
COUNT AS:	4 proteins
	½ fruit

If you're having a hard time getting in all your fruit servings, try fruit chutney or salsa as a topping for meat or fish.

Broiled Salmon with Olive Salsa

1¼-lb salmon fillet, patted dry
⅛ tsp onion powder
SALSA
    2 tsp canola oil
    ½ cup chopped onion
    2 garlic cloves, chopped
    ½ red bell pepper, chopped
    20 pitted small green olives, sliced
    6 sundried tomato pieces, sliced

1 Remove broiler pan; coat pan with nonstick spray. Heat broiler. Measure salmon at thickest part.

2 Place salmon on middle of sprayed rack; sprinkle with onion powder.

3 Broil 10 minutes per in. thickness.

4 Meanwhile prepare Salsa: Heat oil in a medium skillet over medium heat. Add onion and garlic; sauté for 2 minutes. Add red bell pepper; cook 3 minutes. Add olives and sundried tomatoes; simmer on low heat 3 minutes.

5 Serve salsa on salmon.

YIELD:	4 servings
SERVING SIZE:	4 oz
CALORIES:	250
COUNT AS:	4 protein
	1 fat

Salmon contains significant amounts of omega-3 fatty acids, a type of fat that not only helps reduce the risk of heart disease but may also help prevent cancer.

Apricot-Lemon Glazed Fish Fillets

¼ cup apricot spreadable fruit
Juice and pulp of 1 lemon (about 2½ Tbsp)
1¼ lb tilapia fillets (see Note)
⅛ tsp onion powder
2 Tbsp chopped fresh parsley
Salt and pepper

1 Heat oven to 425°F. Spray baking dish with nonstick cooking spray.

2 Place apricot spreadable fruit in small bowl. Squeeze juice and pulp of lemon into bowl and stir to combine.

3 Rinse fish fillets and pat dry. Season lightly with salt, pepper and onion powder.

4 Place fillets in baking pan.

5 Brush apricot mixture on top of fillets.

6 Bake for 10 to 12 minutes, 10 minutes per in. thickness of fillet). Bake until fish is white and flaky.

7 Garnish fish with fresh parsley.

Note: This recipe also works well with cod, scrod, catfish or turbot fillets.

YIELD:	4 servings
SERVING SIZE:	4 oz
CALORIES:	127
COUNT AS:	4 proteins

Pregnant or nursing women and young children should avoid eating tilefish, swordfish, king mackerel and shark, because these types of fish may contain high levels of mercury.

Vegetarian Chili

1 Tbsp canola oil
1 yellow onion, chopped
1 can (28 oz) crushed tomatoes
1 cup sliced carrot
1 cup sliced celery
1 red bell pepper, chopped
1 to 2 tsp minced fresh jalapeno
1 can (19 oz) red kidney beans, drained
    and rinsed
2 cups fully cooked brown rice, wild rice
    or bulgur
Salt and pepper

1 Heat oil in a large saucepan over medium heat. Add onion and cook, stirring occasionally, until tender, about 6 minutes.

2 Stir in tomatoes, carrot, celery, bell pepper and jalapeno and simmer uncovered over low heat for 30 minutes, stirring occasionally.

3 Stir in kidney beans and rice. Continue cooking 5 minutes more until heated through. Season with salt and pepper.

YIELD:	4 servings
SERVING SIZE:	1½ cup
CALORIES:	323
COUNT AS:	3 bread/starches
	2 vegetables
	1 protein

This low-calorie chili has 11 g fiber per serving.

Chicken Vegetable Stir-Fry

MARINADE
    3 Tbsp *each* balsamic vinegar and
        lite soy sauce
    1 Tbsp lemon juice
1¼ lb boneless, skinless chicken breasts,
    cut in 1½-in. chunks
2 tsp olive oil
2 garlic cloves, chopped
2 cups fresh broccoli florets
1 cup baby carrots
4 oz fresh green beans, cut in half (1 cup)
1 red bell pepper, cored and thinly sliced
½ cup water
3 Tbsp flour

1 Mix Marinade ingredients in a shallow bowl. Add chicken, cover and refrigerate at least 2 hours or overnight.

2 Heat oil in a large nonstick skillet; add garlic and sauté until aromatic. Discard marinade and add chicken and brown on all sides.

3 Stir in vegetables, cover and simmer 15 minutes, stirring once or twice.

4 Whisk water and flour in a small bowl until smooth. Add to skillet; stir to mix and coat. Cook over medium heat 2 to 3 minutes until sauce thickens.

YIELD:	4 servings
SERVING SIZE:	1¾ cups
CALORIES:	225
COUNT AS:	4 proteins
	2 vegetables
	½ fat

You can make this stir-fry recipe using shrimp or turkey breast, too.

Bow-Tie Pasta with Beans and Vegetables

QUICK MARINARA SAUCE (SEE NOTE)
1 Tbsp olive oil
½ cup chopped onion
2 garlic cloves, chopped
1 can (28 oz) crushed tomatoes
2 Tbsp tomato paste
½ cup red wine
½ cup chopped fresh parsley or basil,
    plus more for sprinkling
6 oz dry bow-tie pasta
1 cup small broccoli florets
1 cup sliced baby carrots
1 can (19 oz) white beans, drained
    and rinsed
¼ cup grated Parmesan cheese
Garnish: parsley sprigs (optional)

1 Heat oil in medium saucepan over medium heat. Add onion and garlic and cook, stirring, until tender, about 6 minutes.

2 Add tomatoes, paste, parsley and red wine. Simmer over low heat, stirring occasionally, until sauce is thick, about 45 minutes.

3 Cook pasta according to pkg directions.

4 Steam broccoli and carrots until crisp-tender, about 4 minutes.

5 In large bowl combine cooked pasta, steamed vegetables and beans. Toss with desired amount of marinara sauce.

6 Sprinkle 1 Tbsp Parmesan cheese on each serving. Garnish with parsley sprigs, if desired.

Note: Use prepared marinara sauce if you don't have the time to make this.

YIELD:	4 servings
SERVING SIZE:	2 cups
CALORIES:	300 calories (without marinara sauce)
COUNT AS:	2½ bread/starches
	1 protein
	1 fat

This recipe combines pasta (a medium glycemic food) with lots of fiber-rich vegetables and beans, to allow the meal to digest more slowly.

Pear and Chicken Salad

2 cups torn lettuce
1 fresh pear, cut into chunks
1 small cooked chicken breast
    (skin removed), cut into strips
⅓ cup cooked wild rice
2 Tbsp lemon juice
2 tsp olive oil

1 Combine lettuce, pear, chicken and wild rice in a large salad bowl.

2 Whisk together last 2 ingredients; pour over salad and toss lightly.

YIELD:	1 serving
SERVING SIZE:	4 cups
CALORIES:	400
COUNT AS:	3 proteins
	1 fruit
	2 vegetables
	1 bread/starch
	2 fats

Chicken Caesar salad prepared in a restaurant contains twice the calories and three times the fat as this dish. Cook extra chicken and wild rice the night before to have all ingredients handy.

Feta Cheese Wrap

Four 8-in. flour tortillas
DRESSING
    1 Tbsp lemon juice
    2 tsp olive oil
    1 garlic clove, finely chopped
1 cup fresh spinach, cut in strips
1 cup *each* finely chopped cucumber,
    tomato and celery
½ cup shredded carrots
6 oz feta cheese, crumbled
½ cup cooked brown rice
20 pitted black olives: 16 chopped, 4 sliced
    and reserved for garnish (optional)

1 Prepare tortillas as pkg directs.

2 Whisk Dressing ingredients in a large bowl. Add vegetables, cheese, rice and chopped olives; toss to mix and coat.

3 Place tortillas in a single layer on work surface. Spread ¼ of the filling on each. Roll up and secure with a few toothpicks. Garnish each wrap with sliced olives.

YIELD:	4 wraps
SERVING SIZE:	1 wrap
CALORIES:	360
COUNT AS:	1½ proteins
	2 bread/starches
	2 vegetables
	2 fats

Make sure you use 8-in. flour tortillas, rather than the 10- or 12-in. size commonly used in sandwich shops and delis. The larger size will add 80 calories and another bread/starch serving to each wrap.

Tangy Tuna Salad

1 can (6 oz) solid white tuna in water, drained
1 Granny Smith apple, halved and cored
3 whole walnuts, chopped (about 1 Tbsp)
1 Tbsp light mayonnaise
1½ Tbsp chopped onion

Place tuna in small bowl and break into small chunks. Finely chop half the apple. Add to tuna with walnuts, mayonnaise and onion. Stir until blended. Thinly slice remaining ½ apple and use as garnish.

YIELD:	2 servings
SERVING SIZE:	¾ cup
CALORIES:	195
COUNT AS:	3 proteins
	1 fat
	½ fruit

Beware of the tuna salad you buy at your local delicatessen. One scoop may contain as much as 30 g fat!

Lentils with a Twist

1 cup dry lentils
2 cups water
½ cup chopped onion
½ cup chopped celery
2 garlic cloves, chopped
3 Tbsp fresh lime juice
2 Tbsp balsamic vinegar
1½ Tbsp olive oil
2 plum tomatoes, chopped
2 Tbsp chopped fresh cilantro
Salt and pepper

1 Rinse lentils, then place in a medium saucepan with water. Bring to a boil, reduce heat and simmer for 20 minutes, until lentils are tender. Set aside.

2 Meanwhile, spray a large skillet with nonstick cooking spray. Add onion, celery and garlic and cook, stirring, until tender, about 6 minutes. Remove from heat and stir in the lentils, scraping up any brown bits in the bottom of the pan.

3 In a large bowl, whisk together lime juice, vinegar and oil. Add the lentil mixture, tomatoes and cilantro. Season with salt and pepper to taste, and serve warm or cold.

YIELD:	6 servings
SERVING SIZE:	⅔ cup
CALORIES:	170
COUNT AS:	1½ bread/starches
	1 protein

Legumes (dried peas, beans and lentils) are ideal for dieters because they're packed with plant protein, nutrients and fiber.

Wild Rice with Mushrooms and Red Pepper

4 cups water
2 bouillon cubes, any flavor
1 cup dry wild rice
1 Tbsp olive or canola oil
2 garlic cloves, crushed
6 oz small mushrooms, quartered
    (2 cups)
1 red bell pepper, quartered lengthwise
    and thinly sliced crosswise
Salt and pepper

1 Place water, bouillon cubes and wild rice in medium saucepan.

2 Bring to a boil, reduce heat and simmer uncovered until rice is tender, about 55 minutes. (If mixture seems dry before rice is completely cooked, add more water to the pot.) Set aside.

3 Heat oil in a medium skillet. Add garlic, mushrooms and bell pepper and cook, stirring occasionally until tender, about 10 minutes.

4 Stir in wild rice, salt and pepper to taste, and serve hot or cold.

YIELD:	about 6½ servings
SERVING SIZE:	¾ cup
CALORIES:	110
COUNT AS:	1 bread/starch
	½ fat

Wild rice isn't really rice at all, but rather a seed from a tall grass. It contains a good amount of fiber and provides much more protein than white or brown rice.

Sweet Potato Oven Fries

2 medium sweet potatoes (12 oz total), peeled
1 Tbsp plus 1 tsp olive or canola oil
½ tsp paprika
¼ tsp *each* garlic powder, salt and pepper

1 Heat oven to 450°F. Spray a baking sheet with nonstick cooking spray.

2 Cut sweet potatoes into French fries (about 3 in. long and ¼ in. thick), place in a large bowl and toss with oil, paprika, garlic powder, salt and pepper.

3 Arrange sweet potatoes in a single layer on prepared baking sheet.

4 Roast sweet potatoes for about 18 minutes, turning once, until lightly browned and tender. Serve immediately.

YIELD:	4 servings
SERVING SIZE:	3 oz
CALORIES:	125
COUNT AS:	1 bread/starch
	1 fat

Sweet potatoes measure lower on the glycemic index than white potatoes and are rich in beta-carotene.

Red Potatoes with Herbs

1½ lb small red potatoes (about 16)
2 Tbsp olive oil
¼ cup chopped fresh basil
¼ cup fresh parsley
1 Tbsp chopped fresh tarragon
¼ tsp onion powder
Salt and pepper

1 Wash and scrub potatoes and place in a large saucepan with cold salted water to cover. Bring to a boil over high heat. Reduce heat and simmer briskly until potatoes are fork-tender.

2 Drain potatoes, cut into quarters and return to the saucepan.

3 Add oil, basil, parsley, tarragon and onion powder and toss well. Season with salt and pepper to taste, and toss again.

YIELD:	4 servings
SERVING SIZE:	6 oz (about 4 whole potatoes or 16 quarters)
CALORIES:	225
COUNT AS:	2 bread/starches
	1½ fats

Red, or new, potatoes are much lower on the glycemic index than russet potatoes.

Oven Roasted Vegetables

1 cup cauliflower florets
1 cup broccoli florets
1 cup sliced carrots
1 yellow pepper, cut into thick strips
1 small zucchini, quartered lengthwise and
    cut into 1-in. pieces
½ medium onion, thinly sliced
2 garlic cloves, thinly sliced
1 Tbsp plus 2 tsp olive or canola oil
Salt and pepper
Hot sauce (optional)

1 Heat oven to 450°F.

2 Spray baking sheet with nonstick cooking spray.

3 Place all of the vegetables in a large bowl or pan and toss with oil to coat. Season with salt and pepper.

4 Place vegetables on baking sheet in a single layer and place on top oven rack.

5 Roast for 20 minutes, until tender and nicely browned. Serve with hot sauce.

YIELD:	5 servings
SERVING SIZE:	1 cup
CALORIES:	78
COUNT AS:	1 vegetable
	1 fat

The small amount of oil and nontraditional cooking method used here create a dish that will convince even the pickiest eater to finish her veggies.

Green Beans with Chive Cream Sauce

1 Tbsp butter
1 shallot, minced
1 Tbsp flour
½ cup nonfat milk
1 Tbsp fresh chives
1 lb fresh green beans, trimmed
Salt and pepper

1 Melt butter in a medium saucepan over medium-low heat.

2 Add shallot and cook, stirring, until softened, about 5 minutes. Whisk in flour to form a paste; cook, whisking, for 1 minute.

3 Gradually whisk in milk, then cook, whisking, until mixture boils. Stir in chives, and season with salt and pepper.

4 Meanwhile, steam beans until tender, 7 to 8 minutes. Arrange in a serving dish and spoon sauce on top.

YIELD:	4 servings
SERVING SIZE:	1 cup beans with 2 Tbsp sauce
CALORIES:	58
COUNT AS:	1 vegetable
	½ fat

This creamy, low-calorie sauce is a great way to liven up plain steamed vegetables.

Cold Bean Salad

DRESSING
    ¼ cup rice vinegar
    3 Tbsp olive oil
    2 Tbsp lemon juice
1 cup cooked lentils
1 cup *each* canned kidney beans and canned
    chickpeas, rinsed

¼ cup chopped onion
1 cup chopped celery
2 garlic cloves, chopped
16 pitted black olives, sliced in half

1 Whisk Dressing ingredients in a large bowl.

2 Add remaining ingredients to bowl and toss to mix and coat.

3 Refrigerate salad at least 2 hours to allow flavors to blend.

YIELD:	8 servings
SERVING SIZE:	½ cup
CALORIES:	160
COUNT AS:	1 bread/starch
	1 protein
	1 fat

A great alternative to potato salad, this side dish provides 5 g fiber per serving.

Fruit Stuffing

2½ cups water
1 chicken bouillon cube
14-oz bag cubed bread stuffing,
    plain or herbed
1 cup *each* chopped celery and onion
1 Granny Smith apple, not peeled,
    cut in bite-size pieces
⅔ cup (about 14 halves) dried apricots,
    chopped

1 Bring water to boil in a large pot. Add bouillon cube; stir until dissolved. Add stuffing mix and toss lightly with 2 forks to moisten. Stir in remaining ingredients.

2 Coat the bottom of a baking dish with nonstick cooking spray and add stuffing mixture.

3 Bake covered in oven at 325°F, 45 minutes until heated through.

YIELD:	10 servings
SERVING SIZE:	1 cup
CALORIES:	190
COUNT AS:	2 bread/starches
	½ fruit

Traditional stuffing recipes contain a whopping 400 calories per cup. This recipe uses fruit and onion to create a moist stuffing without all the fat and calories.

Tangy Vinaigrette Dressing

¼ cup balsamic or red-wine vinegar
    (or ⅛ cup of each)
7 Tbsp olive oil
1½ Tbsp lemon juice
2 garlic cloves, crushed
2 Tbsp fresh parsley, chopped
1 tsp dried mustard
½ tsp salt
¼ tsp pepper

1 Combine all ingredients in a jar or cruet with a top, and shake to mix.

2 Refrigerate for 1 or more hours to combine flavors before using.

YIELD:	1 cup
SERVING SIZE:	1 Tbsp
CALORIES:	60
COUNT AS:	1 fat

It's wise to make your own salad dressing, since many prepared dressings available contain a lot of sugar.

Tasty Bulgur with Olives and Peppers

2 cups low-sodium chicken broth or water
1 cup dry bulgur wheat
2 tsp olive oil
1 yellow bell pepper, thinly sliced
½ small yellow onion, chopped
2 garlic cloves, minced
1 medium tomato, diced ½ in.
16 black olives, pitted and chopped
Ground pepper

1 Bring water or broth to boil. Rinse bulgur and add to boiling water or broth.

2 Cook, covered, over low heat until all of the liquid is absorbed, 15 to 20 minutes.

3 Meanwhile, heat oil in a large nonstick skillet, add bell pepper, onion and garlic. Cook, stirring, until pepper is softened, about 4 minutes.

4 Add cooked bulgur to skillet and stir to blend flavors. Transfer to a large bowl.

5 Stir in tomato and olives. Season to taste with pepper.

6 Serve warm or cold.

YIELD:	4 servings
SERVING SIZE:	¾ cup
CALORIES:	113
COUNT AS:	1 bread/starch
	1 fat

Bulgur wheat is a healthy Middle-Eastern grain that contains more than twice as much fiber as brown rice.

Flavorful Fruit Crisp

6 cups any combination of seasonal fresh fruit or frozen, unsweetened fruit (apples, cranberries and pears; peaches and blueberries; nectarines and raspberries)
2 tsp lemon juice
TOPPING
    ½ cup whole-wheat flour
    ¼ cup rolled oats
    ¼ cup brown sugar
    ½ Tbsp ground cinnamon
    3 Tbsp cold butter, cut in small pieces
    ¼ cup chopped walnuts
    Pinch of salt

1 Heat oven to 450°F.

2 Prepare fresh fruit: Wash, peel and slice fruit (no need to peel pears or nectarines).

3 Toss together fruit and lemon juice in a shallow 2-quart baking dish (such as a 9 x 13-in. rectangle or a 14-in. oval).

4 Prepare Topping: In a small bowl, mix flour, oats, brown sugar, salt and cinnamon.

5 Cut butter into oat mixture with pastry cutter or two forks.

6 Stir in nuts. Sprinkle Topping over the fruit in the baking dish.

7 Bake 25 to 30 minutes, or until fruit is bubbly and topping begins to brown.

Yield:	6 servings
Serving Size:	¾ cup
Calories:	220
Count As:	2 fruits
	2 fats

Crisps contain much less fat and fewer calories than double-crust fruit pies.

Healthy Chocolate Chip Cookies

½ cup brown sugar
4 Tbsp vegetable oil
4 Tbsp unsalted butter (½ stick)
1 large egg white from 1 large egg
2 tsp vanilla extract
1 cup all-purpose flour
1 cup whole-wheat flour
1 tsp baking soda
¼ tsp salt
¼ cup wheat germ
1 tsp ground cinnamon
½ cup mini chocolate chip morsels

1 Heat oven to 375°F.
2 Have ready 2 large baking sheets.
3 Beat sugar, oil and butter until creamy. Beat in egg, egg white and vanilla.
4 In a separate bowl stir together flours, baking soda, salt, wheat germ and cinnamon.
5 Combine flour mixture with sugar mixture until just blended.
6 Fold in chocolate chips.
7 Shape rounded tsp of dough into disks and place 1 in. apart on baking sheets.
8 Bake for 8 to 10 minutes, until golden.

YIELD:	60 small cookies
SERVING SIZE:	3 cookies
CALORIES:	130 calories
COUNT AS:	1 bread/starch
	1 fat

This recipe uses ½ the fat, ⅓ the sugar and ¼ the chocolate chips found in traditional home-baked chocolate chip cookie recipes. But they' re still delicious!

Yogurt, Lemon and Poppy Seed Bread

1 cup *each* whole-wheat and
    all-purpose flour
2 tsp baking powder
1 tsp baking soda
⅛ tsp salt
¼ cup sugar
1 large egg
1 Tbsp vegetable oil
8 oz (1 cup) nonfat plain yogurt
½ cup nonfat milk
2 tsp lemon extract
1½ Tbsp poppy seeds

1 Heat oven to 350°F. Spray an 8½ x 4¼ x 2½-in. loaf pan (5-cup capacity) with non-stick cooking spray.
2 Mix first 6 ingredients in a large bowl. In a medium bowl, whisk egg, oil, yogurt, milk and extract until blended. Add to flour mixture and stir until just blended. (Don't overmix.) Fold in poppy seeds. Scrape mixture into the prepared pan.
3 Bake 45 minutes or until a pick inserted in center comes out clean. Cool in pan on a wire rack 10 minutes, then remove bread from pan to rack to cool completely.

YIELD:	1 loaf (12 slices)
SERVING SIZE:	1 slice
CALORIES:	105
COUNT AS:	1 bread/starch
	½ fat

Commercially prepared breads and muffins may contain up to 400 calories and 20 g fat per serving. Most store-bought muffins have more than twice the sugar, too!

Mocha Float

1 cup lowfat vanilla yogurt
½ cup nonfat milk
1 large, very ripe banana
3 Tbsp lite chocolate syrup
⅓ cup coffee, decaffeinated or regular
    (left over from the morning pot)
2 tsp vanilla extract
8 ice cubes
½ cup coffee ice cream
    (with no more than 9 g fat per ½ cup)
2 Tbsp fat-free nondairy whipped
    topping (optional)
2 maraschino cherries (optional)

1 Place first 7 ingredients in a blender.
2 Process for 20 seconds or until well blended.
3 Pour into 2 large glasses.
4 Top each with ¼-cup scoop ice cream.
5 If desired, top each float with 1 Tbsp nondairy topping and a maraschino cherry.

Yield:	2 servings
Serving Size:	10 oz
Calories:	280
Count As:	1 dairy
	1 fat
	2 fruits

Beware the mocha coolers prepared at specialty coffee shops. A 12-oz serving can contain as much as 340 calories and 21 g fat.

Apple and Pear Parfait

16 oz (2 cups) nonfat plain yogurt
4 Tbsp apricot spreadable fruit
½ cup frozen nonfat whipped topping,
    thawed
1 McIntosh apple, cored, cut in bite-size pieces
1 pear, cored, cut in bite-size pieces
4 Tbsp chopped walnuts
Garnish: 4 maraschino cherries (optional)

1 To thicken the yogurt, place it in a paper towel–lined strainer set over a bowl or pan to collect the fluid. Let drain in the refrigerator 2 hours.
2 Pour out liquid; transfer solids to bowl. Stir in apricot spreadable fruit.
3 Place ½ the yogurt mixture in 4 parfait glasses. Add ⅓ the whipped topping. Layer with ½ the apple and pear, then ½ the walnuts. Repeat layers once. Spoon on rest of topping; garnish with a cherry.

Yield:	4 servings
Serving Size:	1 parfait
Calories:	175
Count As:	½ dairy
	1 fruit
	1 fat

This low-calorie dessert will add 200 mg to your daily calcium intake.

8. The Tools You Need

YOUR ROAD MAP TO HEALTH

LOSING WEIGHT, IMPROVING YOUR HEALTH and, in the process, changing your outlook on life is a journey. Like all journeys it is best embarked on with a plan—a road map of sorts. This section of the book contains worksheets and logs to guide you through the process of planning, monitoring, troubleshooting and evaluating your progress.

You should make multiple copies of the worksheets before using them. Some records should be kept daily, and others should be used weekly or quarterly. You may find that as time passes your short- and long-term goals change, and you will want to document these changes. During this journey you may change your course or take a detour or, if you're lucky, a short cut. Supply yourself with many worksheets to track and change your plan to meet your needs.

THE PAPER TRAIL

Completing the daily food log will give you immediate feedback on your plan and will increase your awareness of what you're eating every day. The goal worksheet will guide you in laying down the foundation for your newfound plan for health. The emotional eating worksheet will help you pinpoint your specific eating triggers and help redirect your responses to these emotions. Recording your weekly activities on the exercise sheet will guide you in increasing your physical activity level. Finally, don't forget to plot your weight on the weekly weight-loss graph so you can evaluate your progress over time.

DAILY FOOD LOG

DAY _____   DATE _____

TIME	FOOD ITEM	AMOUNT	FOOD CHOICE EXCHANGES

Track food choice exchange totals above, then check off amounts eaten below.

FOOD GROUP	DAILY SERVINGS										+/- TOTALS
Proteins											
Bread/starches											
Fruits											
Vegetables											
Dairy											
Fats											
Water intake	6–8 8-oz glasses										

NOTES _____

DAILY FOOD LOG (Sample)

DAY Wednesday   DATE 1/15/03

TIME	FOOD ITEM	AMOUNT	FOOD CHOICE EXCHANGES
8 A.M.	Whole-wheat English muffin	1 whole	2 bread/starches
	Natural peanut butter	2 tsp	1 fat
	Melon cubes	1 cup	1 fruit
1 P.M.	Lentil soup	1 cup	1 protein and 1 bread/starch
	Whole-wheat melba toast	4 slices	1 bread/starch
	Salad greens	2 cups	2 vegetables
	Vinaigrette dressing	1 Tbsp	1 fat
7 P.M.	Broiled chicken	6 oz	6 proteins
	Sweet potato	one (6 oz)	2 bread/starches
	Steamed spinach	1 cup	2 vegetables
	Salad greens	2 cups	2 vegetables
	Vinaigrette dressing	2 Tbsp	2 fats
	Nonfat milk	8 oz	1 dairy
9 P.M.	Artificially sweetened yogurt	8 oz	1 dairy
	Pear	1	1 fruit

Track food choice exchange totals above, then check off amounts eaten below.

FOOD GROUP	DAILY SERVINGS											+/- TOTALS
Proteins	8	X	X	X	X	X	X	X				-1
Bread/starches	4	X	X	X	X	X	X					+2
Fruits	2	X	X									
Vegetables	4+	X	X	X	X	X	X					+2
Dairy	2	X	X									
Fats	4	X	X	X	X							
Water intake	6–8 8 oz glasses	X	X	X	X							-2

NOTES: I let too many hours lapse between lunch and dinner and was too hungry. I need to drink more water and add more protein, and I should eliminate some of the starches from my menu.

GOAL WORKSHEET

ESTABLISHING A GOAL WEIGHT

DATE

PRESENT WEIGHT

BMI

GOAL WEIGHT

TOTAL POUNDS TO LOSE TO REACH GOAL

% BODY WEIGHT LOSS TO REACH GOAL WEIGHT

BMI FOR GOAL WEIGHT

MAIN GOALS	LONG-TERM PLAN	SHORT-TERM ACTIONS TO SUPPORT LONG-TERM GOALS

COMMENTS:

GOAL WORKSHEET (Sample)

ESTABLISHING A GOAL WEIGHT

DATE	1/15/03
PRESENT WEIGHT	190 pounds
BMI	30
GOAL WEIGHT	155 pounds
TOTAL POUNDS TO LOSE TO REACH GOAL	35 pounds
% BODY WEIGHT LOSS TO REACH GOAL WEIGHT	18%
BMI FOR GOAL WEIGHT	25

MAIN GOALS	LONG-TERM PLAN	SHORT-TERM ACTIONS TO SUPPORT LONG-TERM GOALS
Reach my weight goal	Achieve and maintain a loss of 35 pounds	Follow the diet plan Avoid becoming impatient with any slowdown in weight loss Weigh myself once per week instead of once a day
Exercise more	Maintain a weekly exercise program	Begin a walking program Schedule time to exercise and stick with it.
Reduce my risk of heart disease	Reduce Cholesterol level	Measure fat servings in my meals Increase my fiber intake
Improve my relationship with food	Gain a sense of control over food	Eat small frequent meals to avoid getting too hungry Plan my meals in advance Keep my daily food log

COMMENTS: I am not in a rush to achieve all these important goals. I will not get discouraged if it takes me a while to get where I want to be, as long as I make progress.

EMOTIONAL EATING WORKSHEET

Check off the following emotions that cause you to eat when you aren't hungry. Check all that apply and use the lines to fill in any emotion that is not listed. I EAT WHEN I FEEL:

_____	WORK-RELATED STRESS	_____	I WANT TO CELEBRATE
_____	STRESS AT HOME	_____	ANXIOUS
_____	EXTENDED FAMILY STRESS	_____	LONELY
_____	FINANCIAL STRESS	_____	OVERTIRED
_____	EMOTIONALLY DOWN	_____	BORED

OTHER EMOTIONS THAT MAKE ME OVEREAT:

_____

_____

_____

Make a list of all the things you can do instead of eating to comfort and distract yourself.

1. _____

2. _____

3. _____

4. _____

5. _____

6. _____

7. _____

Be sure to have this list handy when you feel in danger of emotional eating. Post this sheet on the refrigerator as a reminder.

EMOTIONAL EATING WORKSHEET (Sample)

Check off the following emotions that cause you to eat when you aren't hungry. Check all that apply and use the lines to fill in any emotion that is not listed. I EAT WHEN I FEEL:

X	WORK-RELATED STRESS			I WANT TO CELEBRATE
	STRESS AT HOME			ANXIOUS
	EXTENDED FAMILY STRESS		X	LONELY
X	FINANCIAL STRESS			OVERTIRED
X	EMOTIONALLY DOWN		X	BORED

OTHER EMOTIONS THAT MAKE ME OVEREAT:

Feelings of helplessness

Caring for and worrying about my aging parents

Make a list of all the things you can do instead of eating to comfort and distract yourself.

1. Read a book

2. Call a good friend for support

3. Work on my needlework

4. Listen to relaxing music

5. Take a bubble bath

6. Spend time playing with my children

7.

Be sure to have this list handy when you feel in danger of emotional eating. Post this sheet on the refrigerator as a reminder.

PROGRESS REPORT

DATE _____   TOTAL WEIGHT LOST _____

START WEIGHT _____   NUMBER OF POUNDS TO GO
                                       TO REACH GOAL WEIGHT _____
PRESENT WEIGHT _____

HOW I FEEL ABOUT THE PROGRESS I'VE MADE SO FAR:

_____   EXTREMELY HAPPY   _____   VERY HAPPY

_____   SOMEWHAT HAPPY   _____   NOT HAPPY AT ALL

_____   VERY DISAPPOINTED   _____   FRUSTRATED

COMMENTS:
_____
_____
_____

I've experienced these beneficial effects from following the diet and exercise plan.
(Check all that apply to you; use the blank spaces to fill in benefits that are not listed.)

POSITIVE OUTCOME OF MY HEALTHIER DIET AND EXERCISE PLAN	CHECK IF IT APPLIES TO YOU
Increased energy	
Improved self-esteem	
Improved sense of well-being	
Newfound control over food	
Decreased joint pain	
Decreased blood cholesterol level	
Lower blood pressure readings	
Improved sleep habits	
Improved mood	

PROGRESS REPORT (Sample)

DATE   4/15/03   TOTAL WEIGHT LOST   15 pounds

START WEIGHT   190 pounds   NUMBER OF POUNDS TO GO
                                                       TO REACH GOAL WEIGHT   20 pounds
PRESENT WEIGHT   175 pounds

HOW I FEEL ABOUT THE PROGRESS I'VE MADE SO FAR:

_____ EXTREMELY HAPPY   _____ SOMEWHAT HAPPY

_____X_____ VERY HAPPY   _____ NOT HAPPY AT ALL

_____ VERY DISAPPOINTED   _____ FRUSTRATED

COMMENTS:

I had hoped to lose twenty or more pounds by now, but I am happy and feel great. I am trying to
be patient. I know I can follow this diet and exercise plan forever. I'm not hungry and have more
energy than I've had in years.

I've experienced these beneficial effects from following the diet and exercise plan.
(Check all that apply to you; use the blank spaces to fill in benefits that are not listed.)

POSITIVE OUTCOME OF MY HEALTHIER DIET AND EXERCISE PLAN	CHECK IF IT APPLIES TO YOU
Increased energy X	
Improved self-esteem	
Improved sense of well-being X	
Newfound control over food X	
Decreased joint pain	
Decreased blood cholesterol level X	
Lower blood pressure readings	
Improved sleep habits	
Improved mood X	
I don't feel hungry since I'm eating every few hours. X	

LONG-TERM EXERCISE GOALS

MOTIVATION

Please complete the following as a reminder of the factors motivating you to make the **necessary** changes in your exercise routine. Check all comments that apply to you. Add anything **that is** motivating you that is not listed, on the lines provided at the end of this section. It is often **helpful** to review the factors that first motivated you to increase your level of activity whenever **you find** your exercise plan taking a back-seat.

I want to exercise more because:

_____ I WANT TO LOSE WEIGHT

_____ I WANT TO LOWER MY CHOLESTEROL LEVEL

_____ I WANT TO INCREASE MY LEVEL OF ENERGY

_____ I WANT TO LOWER MY BLOOD PRESSURE

_____ I WANT TO GET FIT

_____ I WANT TO FEEL SEXIER

_____ I WANT TO BE ABLE TO KEEP UP WITH MY KIDS

_____ I WANT TO BECOME MORE MUSCULAR

_____ I WANT TO IMPROVE MY HEALTH

_____ I WANT TO IMPROVE MY SPIRITS

_____

_____

_____

_____

FREQUENCY

My long-term goal is to ultimately exercise _____times a week

DURATION

My long-term goal is to ultimately exercise for _____ minutes a session

LONG-TERM EXERCISE GOALS (Sample)

MOTIVATION

Please complete the following as a reminder of the factors motivating you to make the necessary changes in your exercise routine. Check all comments that apply to you. Add anything that is motivating you that is not listed, on the lines provided at the end of this section. It is often helpful to review the factors that first motivated you to increase your level of activity whenever you find your exercise plan taking a back-seat.

I want to exercise more because:

__X__	I WANT TO LOSE WEIGHT	_____	I WANT TO LOWER MY CHOLESTEROL LEVEL
__X__	I WANT TO INCREASE MY LEVEL OF ENERGY	__X__	I WANT TO LOWER MY BLOOD PRESSURE
_____	I WANT TO GET FIT	_____	I WANT TO FEEL SEXIER
_____	I WANT TO BE ABLE TO KEEP UP WITH MY KIDS	__X__	I WANT TO BECOME MORE MUSCULAR
_____	I WANT TO IMPROVE MY HEALTH	__X__	I WANT TO IMPROVE MY SPIRITS

FREQUENCY

My long-term goal is to ultimately exercise _____5_____ times a week

DURATION

My long-term goal is to ultimately exercise for _____45_____ minutes a session

YOUR WEIGHT-LOSS GRAPH

Completing a weight-loss graph will help you monitor and evaluate your progress. A 26-week chart is provided on page 159. Many of my patients monitor their weight in this way for years—even during maintenance. You may want to make copies of this chart for use beyond the 26-week mark. A weight-loss chart will give you a more complete picture of what is happening with your weight. For example, you can evaluate your weight-loss progress monthly or quarterly. Using isolated weekly losses as your measure of progress can set you up for a scary roller-coaster ride. However, seeing your losses plotted on a weekly chart will lay out the big picture for you in black and white.

The numbers across the top of the graph represent the weeks of the program. Week 1 represents the first week of the diet and so on. Along the left side of the graph are numbers representing loss of weight, or gain if that's the case. The change in weight on the left side of the sheet begins with a +4, in case you gain weight before you lose. It doesn't happen often, but sometimes a dieter may actually gain weight before any loss is noted. Poor timing at the start of the diet or gain brought on by fluid retention can be possible causes. If this is the case with you, don't worry, it does not mean that you will not be successful. It means that you need to be patient and keep with the diet. Before you know it you'll be plotting your losses on this chart.

Zero is your starting point. Each square represents two pounds. Place a dot or an X in the box corresponding to the approximate change in your weight under the week you are at in the program. If you take a look at the sample graph, you'll see that this dieter lost 4 pounds in the first week and 2 more pounds in the second, third and fourth weeks of the program—a nice start of 10 pounds lost in the first month. Weeks 9 through 12 tell another story. There's a total loss of only 2 pounds in that month. This dieter gained 6 pounds during weeks 14 through 17 and undoubtedly panicked during that time. Maybe these weeks fell during the winter holiday season or at a time of high family stress. If we evaluate the big picture, however, we see that at the end of 26 weeks this happy dieter lost a total of 38 pounds: an average of about 1½ pounds a week. This graph represents a typical loss curve complete with large losses, weeks of no change in weight and occasional gains. The dieters I care for always seem to have an occasional gain in weight while on this diet. I often see just what the graph shows: bumps in the road, with an overall story of success.

	1	2	3	4	5	6	7	8	9	10	11	12	13	14	15	16	17	18	19	20	21	22	23	24	25	26
+4																										
+2																										
0																										
−2																										
−4																										
−6																										
−8																										
−10																										
−12																										
−14																										
−16																										
−18																										
−20																										
−22																										
−24																										
−26																										
−28																										
−30																										
−32																										
−34																										
−36																										
−38																										
−40																										
−42																										
−44																										
−46																										
−48																										
−50																										
−52																										
−54																										
−56																										
−58																										
−60																										

WEIGHT GRAPH
WEIGHT LOSS VS. WEEKS ON PROGRAM

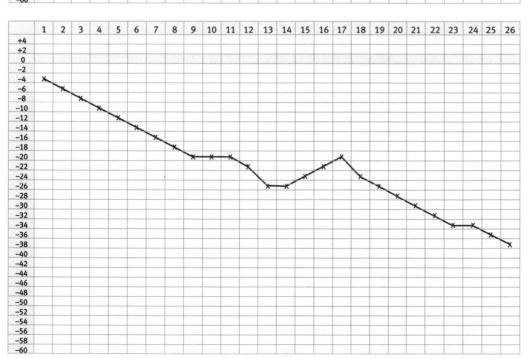

WEIGHT GRAPH (Sample)
WEIGHT LOSS VS. WEEKS ON PROGRAM

16-WEEK EXERCISE LOG

DATE	TYPE OF EXERCISE	MINUTES COMPLETED	COMMENTS

ACKNOWLEDGMENTS

I would like to thank my patients who have generously shared their struggles and successes in the battle to achieve a healthier weight and improve their lives. Their candor and determination has helped me understand what no textbook could describe.

Louis J. Aronne, M.D., deserves my heartfelt gratitude for being an extraordinary instructor and mentor. I've learned volumes about obesity care under his expert guidance. My gratitude extends to Ileana Vargas, M.D., and Judith Korner, M.D.,Ph.D., for their many contributions to my improved understanding of obesity. I'd also like to thank my fellow dietitians, Janet Feinstein, M.S., R.D., and Janice McCabe, M.S., R.D., C.D.E., who continually share their expertise and offer their support. I would also like to thank my good friends and colleagues Deborah Levitt, Ph.D., Nancy Restucci, M.S., R.D., and Karen Speranza, M.S., R.D., who have encouraged me during the development of this book.

I am so very grateful to Donna Behen who gave me my first break in publishing. Donna gives my words clarity and life, and she did just that while editing this entire book. My gratitude extends to Jane Chesnutt, editor-in-chief of *Woman's Day* magazine, for believing in my work, and to her entire staff for their hard work and support.

I consider myself extremely lucky to have published my first book under the superb direction of Dorothée Walliser at Filipacchi Publishing. Many thanks to everyone at Filipacchi who supported my mission and worked so hard to create this wonderful book.

My family lovingly delivered help and encouragement during the writing of this book. My mother, Marion Keenan, encouraged me every step of the way. My brother Robert Keenan and sister-in-law Vivian Fabbro Keenan deserve special mention. Long before I wrote a single word Bob insisted that I could, and should find the time to write this book—and so I did. My sister Marian Engelhardt provided an unending source of encouragement and help. My sister Carol Pinola was the first to suggest that I write for magazines, which launched my writing career, and I will be forever grateful for her foresight. My sister Joanne Keenan Miller and her husband, Jeff Miller, were invaluable in providing feedback and ideas. My sister Lorraine Egan delighted in the production of this book as well. My husband, Fred, and children, Michelle, Brian and Gregory, fueled my daily work engine with love and encouragement. I thank you all.

The publisher wishes to thank Jane Chesnutt and Madonna Behen, Dionisia Colon, Nancy Dell'Aria, Patricia Fabricant, Margaret T. Farley, Michele Fedele, Ellen R. Greene, Jacqueline Hopkins, Sue Kakstys, Gary Krystofiak, Brad Pallas, Karen Quatsoe, Robb Riedel, Greg Robertson, Tony Romano, Stephen Romeo, Tracey Seaman, Marisol Vera and Kim Walker.

SELECTED BIBLIOGRAPHY

It would be impossible to list the hundreds of scientific studies and references used to compile the data in this book. Below are a few selections that were particularly helpful.

The American Dietetic Association—Position Paper. 1999. "Women's Heath and Nutrition-Position of ADA and Dietitians of Canada." *Journal of the American Dietetic Association*, 99: 738–751.

Aronne, L. J. 2001. "Epidemiology, Morbidity and Treatment of Overweight and Obesity." *Journal of Clinical Psychiatry*, 62 Supplement 23: 13–22.

Aronne, L. J. 2001. "Treating Obesity: A New Target for Prevention of Coronary Heart Disease." *Progressive Cardiovascular Nursing*, Summer; 16(3): 98–106.

Brand-Miller, J., Holt, Pawlak and McMillian. 2002. "Glycemic Index and Obesity." *American Journal of Clinical Nutrition*, 76(1): 281S–285S.

Bray, G. 1998. *Contemporary Diagnosis and Management of Obesity.* Pennsylvania: Handbooks in Healthcare, Co.

Cromwell, D. 1995. "Weight Change in the Postpartum Period." *Journal of Nurse-Midwifery*, 40(5): 418–423.

Ewles, A. A. 2002. "Phytoestrogens in the Management of the Menopause: Up-to-Date." *Obstetrical Gynocology Survey*, 57(5): 306–13.

Gunderson, E., and Abrams, B. 2001. "Does the Pattern of Postpartum Weight Change Differ According to Pregravid Body Size?" *International Journal of Obesity*, 25(6): 853–862.

Hamilton, Matvienko, Lewis and Schafer. 2001. "A College Nutrition Science Course as an Intervention to Prevent Weight Gain in Female College Freshmen." *Journal of Nutrition Education*, 33(2); 95–101.

National Institutes of Health. 2000. *The Practical Guide—Identification, Evaluation and Treatment of Overweight and Obesity in Adults.* U.S. Department of Health and Human Services. Publication #00-4084.

Pennington, J. 1998. *Bowes & Church's Food Values of Portions Commonly Used.* New York: Lippincott.

Shils, M. 1994. *Modern Nutrition in Health and Disease—8th edition.* Philadelphia: Lea & Febiger.

Sirtori C. R. 2001. "Risks and Benefits of Soy Phytoestrogens in Cardiovascular Diseases, Cancer, Climacteric Symptoms and Osteoporosis." *Drug Safety*, 24(9): 665–82.

Warshaw, H. 1998. *The American Diabetes Association Guide to Healthy Restaurant Eating.* Alexandria, Va.: The American Diabetes Association.

RESOURCES

General Health and Weight Loss

THE AMERICAN DIETETIC ASSOCIATION
216 W. Jackson Blvd., Suite 700
Chicago, IL 60606
312-899-0040
800-877-1600
800-366-1655 (to find a registered dietitian
   in your area)
www.eatright.org
*Founded in 1917, this is the largest organization of
food and nutrition professionals with almost 70,000
members nationwide. Call or visit the Web site to locate
a qualified health care professional in your area.*

AMERICAN HEART ASSOCIATION
National Center
7272 Greenville Avenue
Dallas, TX 75231
800-AHA-USA-1 (800-242-8721)
www.americanheart.org

AMERICAN DIABETES ASSOCIATION
1701 North Beauregard St.
Alexandria, VA 22311
800-DIABETES (800-342-2383)
www.diabetes.org

**CENTER FOR SCIENCE IN THE
PUBLIC INTEREST**
1875 Connecticut Ave. N.W.
Suite 300
Washington, DC 20009
202-332-9110
www.cspinet.org
*This is a nonprofit public education and advocacy
organization.*

NATIONAL INSTITUTES OF HEALTH
National Heart, Lung and Blood Institute
Education Program Information
P.O. Box 30105
Bethesda, MD 20824-0105
The "Aim for a Healthy Weight" program can be
   found at: www.nhlbi.nih.gov/health/public/
   heart/obesity/lose_wt/index.htm

NATIONAL INSTITUTES OF HEALTH
The Office of Research on Women's Health
   (ORWH)
www4.od.nih.gov/orwh

AMERICAN OBESITY ASSOCIATION
1250 24th St., NW, Suite 300
Washington, DC 20037
www.obesity.org

**NORTH AMERICAN ASSOCIATION FOR THE
STUDY OF OBESITY**
8630 Fenton St., Suite 918
Silver Springs, MD 20910
301-563-6526
www.naaso.org

Eating Disorders

NATIONAL EATING DISORDERS ASSOCIATION
603 Stewart St., Suite 803
Seattle, WA 98101
206-382-3587
www.nationaleatingdisorders.org

**NATIONAL ASSOCIATION OF ANOREXIA
NERVOSA AND ASSOCIATED DISORDERS**
P.O. Box 7
Highland Park, IL 60035
847-831-3438 (hotline)
www.anad.org

INDEX